P.A.C.E.

The 12-Minute Fitness Revolution

Al Sears, MD

Published by:
Wellness Research & Consulting, Inc.
11903 Southern Blvd., Ste. 208
Royal Palm Beach, FL 33411
www.AlSearsMD.com

Warning-Disclaimer: Dr. Al Sears wrote this book to provide information in regard to the subject matter covered. Every effort has been made to make this book as complete and accurate as possible. The purpose of this book is to educate. The author and the publisher shall have neither liability nor responsibility to any person or entity with respect to any loss, damage, or injury caused or alleged to be caused directly or indirectly by the information contained in this book. The information presented herein is in no way intended as a substitute for medical counseling or medical attention.

Copyright © 2010 by **Wellness Research & Consulting, Inc.**
All rights reserved.

Trademark Certification for PACE®
From U.S. Patent Office

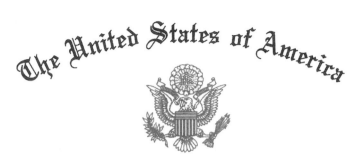

The United States of America

CERTIFICATE OF REGISTRATION
SUPPLEMENTAL REGISTER

Int. Cl.: 41

Prior U.S. Cls.: 100, 101, and 107

Reg. No. 2,950,571

United States Patent and Trademark Office   Registered May 10, 2005

SERVICE MARK
SUPPLEMENTAL REGISTER

PROGRESSIVELY ACCELERATING CARDIOPULMONARY EXERTION

SEARS, AL (UNITED STATES INDIVIDUAL)
12794 W. FOREST HILL BLVD.
WELLINGTON, FL 33414

FOR: PHYSICAL FITNESS INSTRUCTION, NAMELY, DESIGNING EXERCISE PROGRAMS TO PROVIDE CONDITIONING WITHOUT LONG ENDURANCE TRAINING, APPLICABLE WITH A

WIDE VARIETY OF EXERCISE TOOLS, IN CLASS 41 (U.S. CLS. 100, 101 AND 107).

FIRST USE 1-1-2001; IN COMMERCE 5-1-2002.

SER. NO. 76-539,336, FILED P.R. 7-31-2003; AM. S.R. 3-11-2005.

BARBARA BROWN, EXAMINING ATTORNEY

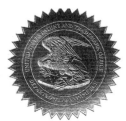

Director of the United States Patent and Trademark Office

Praise for PACE From World-Renowned Doctors

"Dr. Sears blows away the conventional medical wisdom – could it be that cardio training is <u>bad</u> for your health? Dr. Sears makes the impossible seem possible, well written and referenced. If he's right… it changes everything."
Ronald Klatz, MD, DO
Founder and President, American Academy of Anti-Aging Medicine
www.worldhealth.net

"Dr. Al Sears has distinguished himself as a leader in the area of Anti-Aging Medicine and recently in cell and telomere biology.

Now, he boldly introduces the PACE fitness program. This challenges present day exercise theory. However, the program is backed by considerable research, and I predict it will become a standard part of a progressive Anti-Aging Protocol."
Frederic J. Vagnini, MD, FACS; Medical Director of the Heart, Diabetes and Weight Loss Centers of NY

"Unlike any exercise program that's come before it, PACE enables you to get fit and stay fit regardless of where you started. It gives your body the chance to make the changes you need to stay lean, trim and disease-free."
Dr. Lynne Kavulich
Founder and Director of "American Wellness Care"

"If you exercise, you should read this book, and immediately improve the quality of your workout time. If you don't exercise, you should read this book, and start right away on the road to a longer, healthier, more vibrant life."
Frank Shallenberger, MD, HMD, ABAAM
Medical Director, The Nevada Center for Anti-Aging Medicine
Author of *Bursting With Energy* and *The Type 2 Diabetes Breakthrough*

"The current fad of 'cardio' exercise, despite some benefits, is unnatural and may result in harm. PACE is the way to go."
Khalid Mahmud, MD, FACP
Innovative Directions in Health, Minneapolis, MN

"Dr. Sears masterfully explains how we can flip the switches that allow access to the store of human vitality that resides within each one of us. We understood how to do this when we were young and now Dr. Sears gives us the evidence-based means to tap into our potency, strength, and stamina with intention."
Paul L. Hester, MD, MBA

"Dr. Sears has done a fantastic job of not only explaining WHY this exercise approach works, but HOW to do it in simple terms that anyone can apply to their own lifestyle and condition. Get the book, and get moving!"
Ted Cole, MA, DO, CTN, FAAIM, BCIM
Founder, The Cole Center for Healing

"PACE lives up to its name as a 'fitness revolution.' Dr. Sears cuts through much of the health misinformation presented to the public as gospel. He clearly shows why long aerobic workouts are counterproductive and why low-fat, high-carb diets don't lead to weight loss. Read it and improve your fitness level today."
Terry Grossman, MD

"In this terrific manual, Dr. Sears once again takes on the hide-bound myths of the fitness and health establishment and tells it like it is about exercise—what works and what's a waste of time. Brilliant!"
Jonny Bowden, PhD, CNS
Author of *The Most Effective Natural Cures on Earth* and *The Most Effective Ways to Live Longer*

"As a doctor trained in Functional Medicine, Anti-Aging Health, Certified Clinical Nutritionist, Chiropractor and former competitive bodybuilder, I find the principles outlined in Dr. Sears' book refreshingly practical and effective, as well as scientifically sound.

Not only has Dr. Sears formulated PACE from good scientific support, but also he has garnered the information from the personal-practical application of what those of us who've exercised regularly for over 30 years have found works!"
Douglas Husbands, DC, CCN, ABAAHP
www.drhusbands.com

"People who have been inundated with years of 'low fat' diets and 'cardio' exercise plans will really need to be hit over the head with the reasons for change, and Dr. Sears lays those out in no uncertain terms."
Shannon Ginnan, MD
Medical Director, Reveal

"The research about different types of exercise was 'new news' to me, and I found it very interesting. I plan to incorporate these guidelines into my own yoga practice, and I have already begun sharing some of Dr. Sears' exercise information with several clients – it just makes sense!! How wonderful to have access to a dynamic range of exercise without the expense and inconvenience of gym memberships!"
Dani Hudspeth, RN, LMT, CCH, DHom

"As with the first edition of PACE, this new second edition blends the best of the ancient wisdom of our ancestors with modern scientific fact. Al Sears, MD takes on a lot of exercise and medical dogma, comes out swinging and wins the fight for your better health."
Dave Woynarowski, MD

"The accepted medical mantra is to exercise for weight loss – but Dr. Sears crumbles the cardio myth and explains a different approach to exercise. What appears important is the type of exercise needed for fat burning and health. In his book, Dr. Sears explains in detail the science of his PACE program and how simple it is for anyone to achieve athletic wellness and victory over degenerative aging."
Ellie Phillips, DDS
Author of *Kiss Your Dentist Goodbye*
www.CleanWhiteTeeth.com

"Dr. Al Sears' book, PACE: The 12-Minute Fitness Revolution is a much-needed book. Dr. Sears presents compelling evidence that 'cardio' and aerobic exercising are counter-productive to the body. More importantly, Dr. Sears' book tells you how to overcome illness and achieve health by incorporating a simple exercise regimen. I highly recommend this book to anyone who is looking to achieve their optimal health."
David Brownstein, MD
www.drbrownstein.com

Meet Dr. Sears...

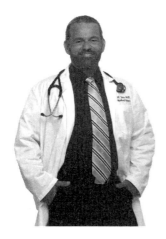

Al Sears, MD is a board-certified medical doctor specializing in alternative and preventative medicine, anti-aging, and nutritional supplementation.

A graduate from the University of South Florida's College of Medicine, Dr. Sears scored in the 99th percentile on his MCAT and graduated with honors in Internal Medicine, Neurology, Psychiatry and Physical Medicine.

His cutting-edge therapies and reputation for solving some of the most difficult-to-diagnose cases attract thousands of patients from around the world to his Health & Wellness Center in Royal Palm Beach, Florida.

As the founder and director of Wellness Research Foundation, a non-profit research organization, Dr. Sears travels the globe to bring back to his patients the latest breakthroughs in natural therapies. Recent trips to Peru, Brazil, India, and Jamaica have yielded important new discoveries in anti-aging and alternative medicine.

One of the first doctors to be board certified in anti-aging medicine, Dr. Sears is an avid researcher, published author and enthusiastic lecturer in the field. He is the first doctor licensed in the U.S. to administer TA-65, arguably the most important breakthrough in anti-aging medicine today.

Dr. Sears is the author of seven books, including *The Doctor's Heart Cure*, and *High Speed Fat Loss in 7 Easy Steps*. He currently writes and publishes the monthly newsletter, *Health Confidential*, and daily email, *Doctor's House Call*, and contributes articles to a host of other publishers in the field. Dr. Sears has appeared on over 50 national radio programs, ABC News, CNN and ESPN.

Professional Memberships

American Medical Association (AMA)
Southern Medical Association (SMA)
American Academy of Anti-Aging Medicine (A4M)
American College of Sports Medicine (ACSM)
American College for the Advancement in Medicine (ACAM)
Herb Research Foundation (HRF)

Certifications

Board certified in anti-aging medicine
Board certified in clinical nutrition
ACE certified fitness trainer

Table of Contents

www.pacerevolution.com

Foreword By
Dr. Jonathan V. Wright, MD

Looking for an exercise program that fits into your busy schedule and really works? You've found it here in Dr. Al Sears' *PACE: The 12-Minute Fitness Revolution*. Even I can fit that into my schedule.

How can 12 minutes a day do what's claimed by this book—rebuild your heart and lung function, and fully activate your body's fat-burning capacity? By following a fundamental principle of good health: Copy Nature! Even better, as Dr. Sears writes, multiple recent research studies are proving that copying "Nature's exercise pattern for humans" is best for your health and mine.

What exactly *is* Nature's exercise pattern for humans? Put briefly, for the majority of humanity's time on Earth, the usual human exercise pattern has been running as fast as possible for only as long as necessary to catch lunch or to avoid being lunch. For the vast majority of human history, weight lifting was done only when there was actual work to do. Few if any individuals did repetitive daily running; cavemen (and cavewomen) didn't go jogging.

Scientific study backs him up. As you'll read in the book, running a marathon creates an inflammatory storm indistinguishable from the early symptoms of heart disease. Dr. Sears cites multiple scientific studies proving that short bursts of intense exercise are best for restoring more youthful lung capacity, lowering cardiovascular risk, and reducing body fat while building muscle.

One of my favorites is Dr. Sears' very own "identical twin study", in which one of the 18-year-old women did the PACE program, and the other did traditional "cardio" exercise. The "cardio" twin ran up to 10 miles a day; the "PACE" twin sprinted 50 yards as fast as she could, rested, and repeated this six times. Although the twins had the same lean body mass and body fat (24.5%) at the beginning of their programs, after 16 weeks, body fat decreased to 10% for the "PACE" twin, while she gained 9 pounds of muscle. The "cardio" exercise twin decreased body fat to 19.5%, and actually lost 2 pounds of muscle.

For me, it's a "no-brainer". Significantly more muscle, significantly less body fat... not to mention lower cardiovascular risk, increased lung capacity... and in a fraction of the time. I know which one I'll choose. I'll copy Nature! How about you?

– Jonathan V. Wright, MD
Medical Director
Tahoma Clinic
Renton, Washington
www.tahomaclinic.com

Author of:
Dr. Wright's Book of Nutritional Therapy (1979) – over 1 million copies sold

And 11 other books, including most recently:
Co-author with Lane Lenard Ph.D. *Why Stomach Acid is Good for You* (2001)
Co-author with Alan R. Gaby M.D. *Natural Medicine, Optimal Wellness* (2006)
Co-author with Lane Lenard, Ph.D. *Stay Young & Sexy with Bio-Identical Hormones* (2010)

Introduction

You and I have a big problem. Unless we do something about it, this problem will make us weak, tired, sick and will probably kill us.

To put it simply, we are not designed for the world we live in. That's our modern predicament.

In the space of a few hundred years, we dramatically changed almost everything about our living conditions. Our world has changed so much in such a short time, we have rendered it unnatural.

As a direct result of these changes, we are in the largest, deadliest and most widespread disease epidemic the world has ever known.

Two out of three Americans are now overweight. Diabetes is nine times more likely than it was just 30 years ago. Heart disease kills over a million people each year in the U.S. alone and, the World Health Organization has recently announced that for the first time in history these modern "chronic diseases" have surpassed all other causes of death worldwide.

Our ancestors evolved to thrive in the world in which they lived. Their daily routines provided them with the physical challenges that kept their bodies lean and muscular.

Being effortlessly energetic with a naturally lean, high-performance body without doing anything conscious to accomplish this is what I call *native fitness*. It's the state of vitality that arises when your body is perfectly matched to your environment. Our ancient ancestors achieved native fitness without thought or effort. It was a natural consequence of their intense struggle to survive.

Now don't misunderstand this observation… ancient life was usually brutal and shortened by high infant mortality, predation and infectious diseases. I'm not suggesting a return to this predator versus prey struggle. But I've studied native cultures around the world. They typically had anatomy and physiology traits we would envy. With strong teeth and bones and lithe bodies, native people were energetic and robust.

In our world we don't have any of the physical challenges that push our heart, lungs and bodies to maximal exertion. And our modern exercise habits fall short to fix this problem.

Our "answers" to inactivity are variations of cardiovascular exercise, jogging, aerobics and weight lifting, all of which are unnatural and ineffective. These so-called solutions just don't provide what our bodies thrived on for millions of years. And far from making us stronger and more resilient, they actually have made us more vulnerable to disease.

As you will learn in the book, these misguided forms of exercise downsize your heart's output, shrink your lungpower and encourage your body to make more fat.

Modern exercise advice has failed you. Enduring hours of drudgery only to increase your risk of disease doesn't make sense. It isn't natural and it doesn't work.

For our ancient ancestors, exertion came in short bouts followed by rest. They didn't run marathons or jump around for an hour at a time without a break. Whether hunting prey, escaping from predators or fighting for their lives, ancient humankind lived in a world where short, intense exertion was followed by periods of rest and recovery.

The body you have right now is a result of this lifestyle. Millions of years of evolution have crafted the heart that's beating in your chest at this very moment. This pattern of brief intensity, followed by rest, is hardwired in your genes.

Your genes define the kind of movement and exertion you need to survive and stay fit. Your muscles, bones and organ systems are reflections of this genetic design. And the way they work together with the challenges of your environment is the formula for strength, vitality and long life.

The trigger that makes it happen is short bursts of exertion followed by rest and recovery.

This natural rhythm produces:

- Expanded lung volume.
- High-speed fat loss.
- Reserve capacity in your heart.
- A higher metabolic rate with increased insulin sensitivity.
- New muscle growth and stronger bones.
- Better sexual performance.

A small group of astute exercise and health professionals have come to the same conclusion: what we need to recondition our bodies and reclaim our native health is short bursts of high intensity intervals. But how?

The average person can't go out and perform at a high intensity for any "interval." As you will learn, these interval training programs are really only adequate for highly conditioned athletes. What about the people who need it most?

PACE is the only system ever designed to safely and effectively recondition our average modern bodies back to optimal fitness. By starting off easy then gradually and incrementally focusing on the right changes, we recreate the challenges of our ideal natural environment. Our bodies are already programmed and perfectly equipped to respond to these challenges. The result is *total health*, not just fat loss or a stronger heart. PACE is a clear path that re-aligns your modern mind and body with the instincts and rhythms of your ancient past.

PACE reawakens your native fitness.

In an ideal world you wouldn't need to exercise. But those days are gone. Today you must act. You must do *something*.

PACE is the answer and the action.

PACE is a growing revolution. It's already practiced by thousands of people in dozens of countries around the world.

PACE overturns years of failed ideas and exercise advice. PACE upends current exercise trends by revealing their flaws and offering a more effective, more natural way of moving our bodies.

The PACE revolution leads us back to ancient times when our bodies were perfectly matched to our environment, to a time when obesity, heart disease and cancer rarely existed.

This book will show you how to replace the flawed and

ineffective theories that have been mistakenly accepted without proof of what really works.

In a matter of weeks, you'll:

- Build strength and reserve capacity in your heart and lungs.
- Avoid heart attacks and cardiovascular disease.
- Develop a powerful and disease-resistant immune system.
- Dramatically increase your energy levels.
- Burn fat, even while you rest.

Join the PACE revolution and your body will soon become naturally strong and resilient. You'll join the cutting-edge group of thousands who now feel energized, motivated and ready to take on any challenge. Your muscles will be their intended size, no bigger or smaller. Your chest will be robust, your waist thin and your breath will be deep and focused.

And the best news is that joining the PACE revolution takes, on average, only 12 minutes per day.

Awaken the dormant, super-fit native inside you. Native fitness is your birthright.

Join me now as we reawaken this vitality.

It's rightfully yours.

To Your Good Health,

Al Sears M.D.

Al Sears, MD

CHAPTER ONE

Are Your Lungs Dying?

It's the Most Destructive Effect of Aging...

I bet your doctor never told you this: As you age, cells in your lungs start to die off faster than you replace them, causing your lungs to shrink.

That's bad news not just for your strength and stamina but also for your ability to fight off disease. And here's the real eye-opener: The smaller your lungs, the greater your chance of dying – *of all causes.*

The groundbreaking Framingham Heart Study looked at data stretching back six decades and concluded your lungs tell you how long you'll live. This ongoing research is particularly convincing for two reasons: it's the longest running study in medical history and it has no involvement from the big drug companies.

Doctors involved in the Framingham Study, William B. Kannel and Helen Hubert, both from the Boston School of Medicine concluded: ***your lungs are the number one predictor of death.***

To put another piece of this monumental discovery in their own words, here's what they said:

"This pulmonary function measurement appears to be an indicator of general health and vigor and *literally a measure of living*

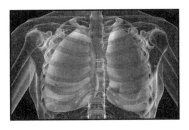

capacity… Long before a person becomes terminally ill, vital capacity can predict life span. The Framingham examinations' predictive powers were as accurate over the 30-year period as were more recent exams."[1]

That's a remarkable equation: Your ability to breathe equals your ability to live.

You won't hear that from your doctor and you won't read about it in the newspaper. But you **can** do something about it. And, your life depends on it.

Have a look at this graph:

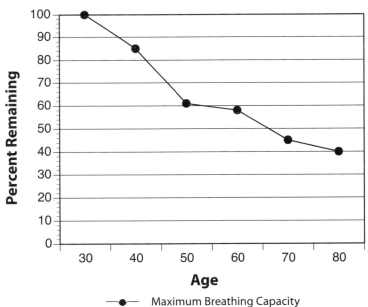

Age Related Loss of Lung Function

—●— Maximum Breathing Capacity

Adapted from "Biological Aging Measurement." Dr. Dean Ward. 1988

More Revelations From the Framingham Heart Study:

Reduced Lung Function Predicts Congestive Heart Failure

Following 5,209 people over 18 years, researchers discovered that the risk of congestive heart failure goes up 10-fold as lungpower decreases. What's more, the people in the study showed no sign of heart disease when their lungpower started to shrink. But as the years went by, those who had smaller lung capacity had up to a 1,000 percent greater chance of developing congestive heart failure.

Here's a quote from the study:

> *"Examination of the net contribution of vital capacity (a measure of lung function) to risk of congestive heart failure revealed that a low vital capacity was associated with development of congestive heart failure even after taking into account other contributing factors including blood pressure, relative weight, pulse rate, cigarette smoking, heart enlargement on X-ray, ECG-LVH, blood glucose and age.* **Both a persistently low and recent fall in vital capacity** *[lungpower]* **were associated with increased risk of congestive heart failure.***"*

This study was published back in 1974... in the prestigious journal of the American Heart Association, Circulation. Yet 35 years later, the medical mainstream still ignores the power of the lungs to predict disease.

Don't wait another day. Put PACE to work for you right now. Just a half hour a week could mean the difference between a heart attack and a healthy, disease-free life.

Kannel WB, Seidman, JM, Fercho, W, Castelli, WP. Vital Capacity and Congestive Heart Failure: The Framingham Study. *Circulation*. 1974;49(6):1160-1166.

By the time you're 50 years old, 40 percent of your lungpower is gone. By the time you're 80, you lose over 60 percent – and that's just an average.

The Framingham Study found your lungpower drops 9 to 27 percent per decade. If you're on the high end of that scale you could lose 80 to 90 percent by the time you retire. Don't expect much help from mainstream medicine. Dr. Kannel and Dr. Hubert announced their findings back in the early 1980s. Yet doctors and the media continue to overlook or ignore this critical breakthrough.

If the Framingham Study were the only one to make this point, it might be easier to understand. But it's not. More recent studies confirm your lungs' ability to predict lifespan and risk of disease.

In 2000, the American College of Chest Physicians published a 29-year follow up to an earlier study from the University of Buffalo. The researchers, led by Dr. Holger J. Schunemann, tested the predictive value of lungpower in both men and women after 29 years. The results were consistent... and sobering.

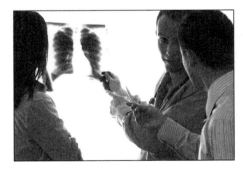

In addition to confirming the link between lungpower and death, they also found an increased risk of death for people with *moderately* impaired lungpower – not just the people who had the worst damage.

Dr. Schunemann remarked, *"It is surprising that this simple measurement has not gained more importance as a general health assessment tool."*[2]

That's quite an understatement.

Your lungpower is the primary predictor of your health and your future. Even if you have just a moderate loss, which most people do, you're at risk.

A pulmonary function test is a tool every doctor should be using. In my own practice I monitor my patients' lungpower and give them simple, easy-to-follow steps to rebuild lost lung capacity. You'll find those techniques in this book.

It's Not Too Late to Stop the Loss... Rebuild Your Lungs and Enjoy the Energy of a 30-Year Old

If you do nothing, you will quickly lose precious lungpower. And with that loss your risk of disease and early death will skyrocket.

If you ask your doctor, they will probably tell you lungpower is not important. What's more, they will tell you it's impossible to maintain or increase your lung capacity. But that's not true. It may be accepted as "fact," but your lungs are not helpless. They respond to the right challenge. In the same way you can build real heart strength, you can build healthy, robust lungs.

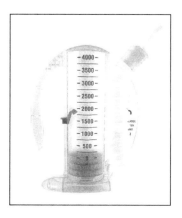

I'm living proof. As of this writing I am 53 and have the lungpower of an 18-year old. This has been verified using independent labs with the latest maximum lungpower-testing technology. I accomplished this simply by following PACE.

Small Lungs Boost Risk of Heart Disease – Even in Young Adults...

The University of Otago in New Zealand discovered a link between reduced lungpower, inflammation and the risk of heart disease.

Measurements of lungpower and blood inflammation were taken when the study participants were 26 years old, and then again when they were 32 years old.

Researchers found higher levels of a key marker of inflammation – C-reactive protein (CRP) – in the blood of those with smaller lungs.

CRP is a risk factor that leads to heart attack, stroke and atherosclerosis (hardening of the arteries).

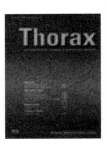

The study's co-author, Dr. Bob Hancox said, *"Increased levels of inflammation markers have previously been found in older people with reduced lung function and chronic obstructive pulmonary disease (COPD), but as far as we know, this is the first time it has been reported in young adults without lung disease."*

In other words, reduced lungpower is related to inflammation. And inflammation leads to heart disease and stroke.

The evidence is clear: the damage starts when you're in your 20s and 30s.

PACE is the only program designed to build lungpower and eliminate the risk of heart attack and stroke associated with inflammation.

Hancox RJ, Poulton R, Green JM, et al. Systemic inflammation and lung function in young adults. *Thorax*. 2007;62(12):1064-1068.

I first observed and documented lungpower when I was an undergraduate in college. I always wanted to be a gymnast but I wasn't that good in tumbling routines. But I could do the strength moves better than anyone on the team.

The coach asked me what weight lifting routine I used to develop shoulder, arm and back strength. When I told him that I didn't lift weights he asked me to assist in strength training the team. I had a job at the school infirmary so I borrowed their equipment to measure as many parameters of strength that I could. This would be our starting point.

As part of this assessment, I ran a series of pulmonary function tests. I put those with the lowest lung volumes into running programs because everyone "knew" that long distance running would make you develop more lungpower, right?

A few months later, after they had finished a long-duration cardio program, I ran another series of lung capacity tests. Much to my initial shock, their lungpower had shrunk. That's when it all began to click…

If you don't challenge your lungs' maximum power you'll actually give up lungpower. What's more, the strain of lost lungpower speeds up the aging process, making you even more vulnerable to infection and chronic disease.

PACE *challenges* your peak lung volume. Short bursts of intense exertion followed by rest send a signal to your lungs to expand. Over time, your body adapts to the challenge by increasing its lung volume and power.

I do the same for my patients. I've helped people across the board. Whether they're recovering smokers, have problems like emphysema or COPD, or simply have a moderate loss of lung function, PACE successfully rebuilds their lungs and gives them greater energy, stamina and performance power.

I have proof that even if you are in your 70s it's still possible to regain and maintain the lung capacity of someone in their 30s. Starting in the late 1960s, the German physicist and inventor Manfred von Ardenne tested the relationship between exercise and lung function.

In one set of studies von Ardenne showed the average loss of lungpower over time. But he also measured the lungpower of older men and women who used one of the techniques in my PACE program – *short bursts of intense exertion followed by rest and recovery.*

He discovered that people who challenge their lungs with the right type of exertion could have the lungpower of someone much younger. This graph reveals his findings:

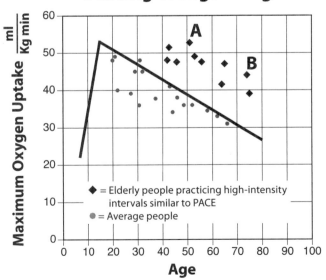

Building Younger Lungs

Adapted from: von Ardenne, M. *Oxygen Multistep Therapy.*
Thieme. 1990. p. 31

www.pacerevolution.com

You can see that maximal oxygen uptake starts to drop off in your 20s and falls sharply as you age. This loss over time is represented by the black line. By the time you're 80, you have lost almost 60 percent of your lungpower.

But the people who challenged their lungs *had younger lungs*. Even in spite of their age. In one example, a man in his early 50s had the lungpower of a 20-year-old (Point A). Another man in his early 70s maintained the power of a 30-year-old (Point B).

Overall, the men who exercised had younger lungs (diamonds) compared to the people who didn't (circles).

Rebuilding your lungs is not only possible, you can do it successfully with little effort. And the benefits go far beyond your lungs.

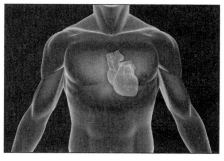

Manfred von Ardenne discovered that your cells produce more energy when you practice short bursts of intense exertion – a capacity you build with my PACE program. This improves the way your organs use oxygen, keeping them younger longer. By keeping your routine focused on short, intense bursts you mimic the movements of our ancient ancestors. And you send waves of life-giving oxygen through every cell in your body.

For thousands of years our hunter-gatherer ancestors stayed fit from activities that involved intense exertion followed by rest. This included hunting, foraging and escaping from wild animals.

Aside from keeping them lean and muscular, this pattern of exertion followed by rest flooded their bodies with oxygen.

Have a look at this table:

Your Blood Flow at Different Levels of Exertion				
Blood Flow (ml/min)				
	Rest	Light Exertion	Heavy Exertion	Maximal Exertion
Brain	750	880	1,000	1,400
Coronary	250	350	750	1,100
Lungs	Basic Value, (BV)	1.4 x BV	3 x BV	4 x BV
Skeletal Muscle	1,200	4,500	12,500	22,000
Cardiac Output	5,800	9,500	17,500	25,000

Adapted from: von Ardenne M. *Oxygen Multistep Therapy*. Thieme. 1990. p. 144

This table shows how blood circulation increases with exertion. The numbers are stunning.

When you look at "maximal exertion," a capacity you achieve from your PACE routine, circulation – and therefore oxygen transport – goes through the roof.

Blood flow to your lungs and your cardiac output increase by *more than 400 percent*. Compare that to the relatively small increases during light exertion, the kind of exertion level you achieve when you practice a medium-intensity challenge like aerobics or cardio.

The difference is important. Your brain gets almost *twice as much blood and oxygen* during maximal exertion than it does with light or medium exertion.

Traditional exercise has failed you. By not recognizing the rate of blood flow associated with different levels of exertion, aerobics and cardio miss the point. And, you won't build your lungs by training for endurance, or by jumping around for an hour while you watch a Richard Simmons workout video.

You build your lungs by challenging their maximal capacity. In other words, you give it everything you have for a very short period of time. Then you rest. What could be simpler?

Why Didn't Anyone Tell You This Before?

Medical students don't learn much about breathing. One study of med students in the UK found they weren't able to reliably tell the difference between normal and abnormal breathing. This, of course, led to a *"high number of inappropriate and potentially harmful actions."*[3]

It's a serious situation. Your lungs are your number one predictor of death, yet most doctors have no clue. Some would even laugh at the idea. And if you're lucky enough to find out, there's no one to turn to… no one to point you in the right direction on what to do about it.

Your lungs are ignored. Modern exercise strategies leave them out completely. No one says anything about them until disease strikes. And by then it's often too late.

Aerobics, cardio and long-distance running are all designed to give your heart more "endurance." That sounds great, except that your body was not designed for the kind of medium-intensity, long-duration activity you get when you practice cardio or aerobics.

Can you think of a situation when cavemen needed to run for hours on end? Or jump around, working up a sweat, repeating the same body movement over and over with no break or rest?

Ancient man had no application, no need and no context for continuous exertion without rest. It was not a part of their daily routine. And that's a critical observation. The body you have right now is a direct result of thousands of years of collective movement and evolution – refined over 100,000 generations.

Your heart and lungs were designed for short bursts of intense exertion followed by rest. And that's the exact opposite of what modern "fitness gurus" tell us to do.

It's the same in the animal kingdom. Animals instinctually exert themselves in small bursts followed by rest. You will very rarely see animals run for hours on end. That kind of movement is not the daily norm in nature.

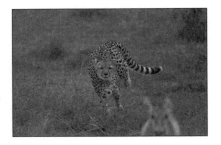

Your lungs need to be challenged to their maximum capacity in order to thrive and stay healthy. Think for a moment… when was the last time you ran as fast as you could? It's probably been a while. Cardio is designed so that you plod along, never running too fast, never running too slow. But what is the purpose?

In ancient times, different forms of quick acceleration (like sprinting) were essential. And this kind of activity, whether on land, or in water, challenged the lungpower of our ancestors.

Check out the graph on the next page.

The middle section – where you see the short, wavy lines – is your normal, everyday breathing. It's called "tidal breathing." Notice it's a very narrow band. Tidal breathing only represents a small fraction of our total lung capacity.

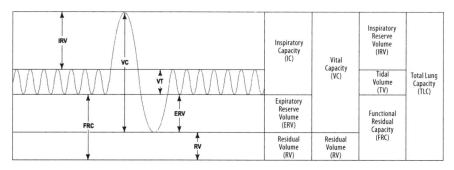

Adapted from the standard output of a spirometer.

In the middle of that, you see one bigger wave. Inside that bigger wave are the letters "VC." That wider band represents your vital capacity. Vital capacity is what shrinks as you age.

Doesn't it make sense that if you want to preserve your lung's vital capacity you need to challenge it? Of course, right? But we never do.

During the course of our busy days, our breathing stays within that narrow band of tidal breathing. And if you go to the gym or practice cardio, your breathing will expand – but you never challenge your vital capacity. And you almost never reach total lung capacity.

Here's what we face: Our vital capacity drops quickly with age. And during the course of our lives we do nothing to change that. In fact, most of us never experience what it's like to breathe fully.

Adding fuel to the fire, day-to-day stress makes breathing short and shallow. Have you ever noticed that you tend to hold your breath when you're tense or stressed out?

A study from Harvard, published in the medical journal *Thorax*, found a connection between anger and decreased lung function.

In the article, Dr. Rosalind Wright of the Harvard School of

Public Health stated, *"hostility is associated with poorer pulmonary function and more rapid rates of decline among older men."*[4]

Modern life is stressful and our lungs take a beating. Often times you don't even realize you're not using them to the fullest – or that you can't.

Loss of lungpower is common and chronic. That means it's a constant problem that continues over many years. You don't notice because you don't have anything to compare it to.

PACE is different. It's the only effective program designed to rebuild and restore your lost lungpower. And it doesn't take more than 12 minutes a day, three times a week.

Obesity Puts Some in Death Spiral

Doctors discovered that obesity restricts a person's lungpower by as much as 20 to 30 percent.

The extra weight pushing on their chest and lungs creates a respiratory resistance that must be overcome in order to breathe.

By increasing the normal loss of lungpower that comes with age, obesity accelerates the aging process and puts people at a higher risk of other chronic diseases, which in turn diminishes the lungs' vital capacity.

PACE not only reverses loss of lungpower, it activates your "native fat burner." In later chapters you will learn how some of my patients lost as much as 18 pounds in a single month.

Zerah F, Harf A, Perlemuter L, Lorino H, Lorino AM, Atlan G. Effects of Obesity on Respiratory Resistance. *Chest.* 1993;103(5):1470-1476.

Supercharge Your Performance by Racking Up an Oxygen Debt

The *oxygen debt* triggers bigger lungs and more lungpower. It happens when your body needs more oxygen than you can give it… like after a short burst of intense exertion. It's one of the key features of PACE.

Conventional wisdom tells you to exercise at a *moderate intensity.* They call this your "aerobic zone." But staying within this narrow band never challenges your limits.

When you do a high-intensity activity – which becomes easy with PACE – you challenge those limits. Once you cross over from medium exertion to intense exertion, you need more and more oxygen to sustain that high level of activity. Sprinting would be a good example. Of course, you can't sprint for very long. You will be exhausted after half a minute or so.

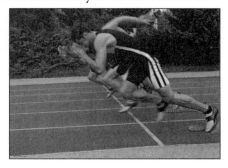

But when you stop sprinting, you'll become short of breath and pant. This is your body's way of getting oxygen back into your body as quickly as possible. The concept is easy to understand: High-intensity activities need lots of oxygen fast.

Oxygen is the basic fuel your cells need to keep moving. When you're jogging, your body can inhale enough oxygen to keep that activity going for quite a while. But when you're sprinting fast, the demand for oxygen is so intense you can't go for even a minute. As you approach maximal exertion, the amount of oxygen required to keep you going will exceed the amount you're taking in – that's the point when you begin accumulating an oxygen debt.

You may wonder why an oxygen debt is important. You might even think that pushing your body to that point is counter-intuitive. After all, why would you want to starve your body of oxygen?

The answer lies in your body's "adaptive response."

Think about what those words mean for a moment… an adaptive response is a change your body makes after confronting a challenge. If you don't give your body new challenges, it won't make these changes. In other words, you won't grow or progress.

That's one of the reasons why aerobics, cardio and long-distance running are not the best options for your long-term health. No progress will be made to build back lung capacity because you are not challenging your current lung capacity. In fact, because you are "preprogrammed" to lose capacity with age, if you don't train your body to make changes in response to challenges, you'll actually start sliding backwards.

But when you give up these long, boring workouts, you can change your body's experience with exertion.

When you achieve oxygen debt, your body responds. Plateaus are broken. Changes are made. First and foremost, your body reacts by increasing your lung volume and boosting your heart's output.

By doing those kind of activities you actually "ask" your body to make those changes. And in response, it does. You can train your body to make any kind of change you want. If you want small, tight lungs and decreased cardiac output, then keep jogging.

But if you want the kind of longevity and heart attack prevention that comes with bigger lungs and a stronger heart, then shoot for an oxygen debt each time you do an exertion period with PACE.

Even a Moderate Drop in Lungpower Increases Your Risk of Heart Attack by Over 200 Percent

Researchers at the Royal Free Hospital School of Medicine in London, in a 7.5 year follow up of 7,735 men, discovered those with even a moderate loss of lungpower had a more than two-fold increase in heart attack risk.

Even after adjustments for other risk factors, including smoking, the increased risk was still over 200 percent.

Their findings were published in the *European Heart Journal*.

Cook DG, Shaper AG. Breathlessness, lung function and the risk of heart attack. *European Heart Journal*. 1988;9(11):1215-1222.

Here's an easy example:

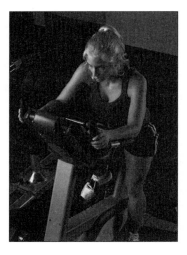

Let's say you're on a stationary bike and you've cranked up the resistance level... enough to give you a considerable challenge.

After a few minutes, your breathing will change. You will need to breathe more deeply and more quickly to sustain that level of intensity. When this happens, pay attention. Instead of breathing with no thought or intention, put some focus on your breath.

When you inhale, do it quickly and fully. Imagine your lungs filling up on both sides of your chest. Both in front and in back. Think of your lungs as two big barrels that fill up quickly all around.

Then exhale quickly and fully. Imagine those barrels depleting – like two dried up raisins.

Repeat this process quickly and steadily. Inhale fully. Exhale fully. Count it off… One, two. One, two. Get into a rhythm and be completely aware of each breath.

In order for you to sustain a high-intensity activity, you have to gain control over your breath. And when you're in the heat of the moment, your breathing needs to be fast and full. No hanging on. No resistance. Give in to it and let go.

Of course, every high-intensity exercise is short lived. And even after focusing on an intense breathing routine, you'll have to stop after a few minutes. But when you do, be very aware of that moment.

From that regulated, fast in, fast out, breathing, you'll stop your activity and break into a pant. The rhythm of your breath will change. The panting will be faster and feel more desperate and out of control.

You can achieve this during any kind of high-intensity activity. It doesn't have to be sprinting or cycling on a stationary bike. It could be anything. Even fast walking.

The key is self-awareness and observation. Watch yourself. As you start to exert yourself, pay attention to your breath. As your breath accelerates, get into a rhythm you can follow. Regulate your breath. And by that I mean allowing yourself to inhale and exhale fully in a repetitive and consistent manner. When you're pushing yourself during PACE, that regulated breathing will be fast and deep. And if you follow these simple guidelines, you can achieve it every time.

Rebuilding your lungs is not impossible. Using the oxygen debt is a surefire way to regain the power, flexibility and stamina of your younger days. It's one of the techniques I use to keep the lung capacity of a 20-year-old. You can do it too.

As you read to the end of your PACE book I will talk about the oxygen debt in more detail. And I'll show you exactly how to use it.

First, let's throw out another popular exercise myth… the misguided notion that jogging, cardio and marathon running are "good" for your heart.

Endnotes

1 Miller, JA. "Making Old Age Measure Up," *Aging*. Vol. 2, Art. 12. Boca Raton, FL.: Social Issues Resource Series, Inc., 1981.

2 Schunemann H. Dorn J, Grant BJ, Winkelstein W Jr, Trevisan M. Pulmonary Function is a Long-term Predictor of Mortality in the General Population. *Chest*. 2000;118(3);656-664.

3 Perkins GD, Stephenson B, Hulme J, Monsieurs KG. Birmingham assessment of breathing study (BABS). *Resuscitation*. 2005;64(1):109-113.

4 Kubzasky LD. Angry breathing: a prospective study of hostility and lung function. *Thorax* 2006;61:863-868.

PACE Success Stories:

"PACE is awesome! I've been overweight most of my adult life and nothing I've tried works. Diets, exercise programs, you name it, I've tried it. I never lost weight, no matter how much I jazzercised, walked, or sweated to the oldies. My body fat is the most stubborn you'll ever imagine. Responds to nothing!

PACE gave me visible results in 2 weeks. That's right, 2 weeks! I thought maybe it was just wishful thinking on my part, until my husband touched me and said, 'Wow, you feel different. You have a waist!'

I'm in my 6th week of PACE, and I'm wearing clothes I'd given up all hope of ever wearing again. People keep asking me what I'm doing and I can't say enough about PACE.

Did I mention I'm a cardiac patient with a pacemaker? I feel better than I have in years, and the best part is, I'm in and out of the gym in a few minutes! I used to spend hours there!

When I think of the thousands of dollars I've spent on their weight loss solutions that were, in reality, no solution, I could cry. Who would have thought it could be this simple?"

Denise B., Alpharetta, GA

෨෴

"Since I have been doing PACE, I feel my body-fat percentage has gone down and my wind and stamina are a lot better. I really feel like you can max-out your aerobic workout in a short amount of time. I would recommend PACE highly to anyone."

Stephen W., Bremen, IN

CHAPTER TWO

Throw Away Your Jogging Shoes

Go to the book store and you'll see magazine covers loaded with creative ways to frame the same advice: You need "cardio." Go to any gym and the trainer will devote some of your workout to "cardio." You probably don't like it, but you feel like you have to go along with it. After all, who doesn't want a healthy heart?

We accept the term "cardio" (short for cardiovascular endurance training or CVE) as a synonym for heart conditioning. Yet when you study the heart's reaction to repeated sessions of cardio, it raises serious concerns.

First, it doesn't really strengthen the heart because endurance and strength are two separate things induced by opposite exercises. Second, this type of continuous challenge simulates episodes of prolonged stress from our once-native hunter environment. It induces short-term survival strategies. But if you stay in survival mode too long it's very destructive.

After 30 years of working with extremely fit athletes, patients with failed, diseased or injured hearts and average people in between, one thing is apparent: doing continuous cardio exercise is a waste of time.

It just doesn't build what your heart needs. It doesn't increase your heart's ability to respond to real demands. In fact, for all your effort, you only *reduce* your ability to handle life's stressful circumstances – the last thing you want.

Yet for decades now, you've heard this advice from nearly every public agency with anything to say about health. The American Medical Association, The Institutes of Medicine, even the new food pyramid from the USDA all focus on durational exercise.

But if you look at the science, it backs me up on an opposite point of view.

For starters, the Harvard Health Professionals Study followed over 7,000 people and found that the key to exercise is NOT length or endurance. It's *intensity.* The more intense the exertion, the lower their risk of heart disease.[1]

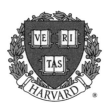

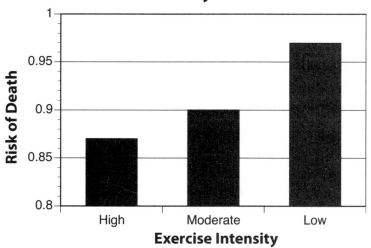

Exercise Intensity and Risk of Death

High intensity exercise is also safer. A separate Harvard study compared vigorous and light exercise.

Those who performed exercise that is more vigorous had a lower risk of death than those who performed less vigorous exercise.[2]

Aerobics, jogging and marathon running are low-intensity, long-duration exercises. The Harvard study clearly shows that this kind of exercise *increases* your risk of heart disease and death.

And here's why: When you exercise for long periods at a low to medium intensity, you train your heart and lungs to get smaller in order to conserve energy and increase efficiency at low intensity.

Yet we are constantly made to feel that if we could just overcome our laziness and make ourselves do enough of this boring drudgery, it would solve our health problems and protect our hearts. If this were true, why do very "conditioned" endurance runners drop dead of heart attacks at the height of their running careers?

Unfortunately, this phenomenon has a 2,500-year history. In ancient Greece, the very first marathon runner dropped dead after his historic 26.2-mile run. As a soldier and messenger, Phidippides ran from the ancient city of Marathon to Athens to announce the victory of the Greeks over the invading Persians. As soon as he yelled, "Nike!" (Victory!), he collapsed and died.

Twenty years ago, I provided emergency care for marathon races. I was surprised to see a thin young man collapse to the ground just yards from our emergency aid station. His heart continued to violently race, as we put an oxygen mask over his blue lips. Another runner in his 20s made it to our station but had to kneel down to wait for emergency assistance. He was weak, dizzy and frightened – with a dangerously irregular heartbeat.

The New York Times Publishes
Clinical Research Supporting PACE

In their article "A Healthy Mix of Rest and Motion," *The New York Times* highlights the effectiveness of the PACE principle *intensity*. The clinical research used for their story was published in the *Journal of Applied Physiology*.

Exercise scientists from the University of Guelph in Ontario proved interval training boosts fat burning, circulation and cardiopulmonary output.

Here's a quote from the article: **The New York Times**

"After interval training, the amount of fat burned in an hour of continuous moderate cycling increased by 36 percent, said Jason L. Talanian, the lead author of the study and an exercise scientist at the University of Guelph in Ontario. Cardiovascular fitness – the ability of the heart and lungs to supply oxygen to working muscles – improved by 13 percent.

It didn't matter how fit the subjects were before. Borderline sedentary subjects and the college athletes had similar increases in fitness and fat burning. 'Even when interval training was added on top of other exercise they were doing, they still saw a significant improvement,' Mr. Talanian said."

Interval training has been around for years and it's far more effective than cardio, aerobics or long-distance running. **But PACE is NOT interval training.**

While interval training is better than typical cardio, it is still a fixed routine. It doesn't focus on the most important element of progression and it doesn't "train" your adaptive responses. So in

(Continued on the next page…)

(Continued from the previous page…)

many ways, interval training has the same problems and pitfalls as aerobics or cardio. And it's difficult for beginners. In fact, most people just can't perform at high intensity intervals.

When you combine the proven benefits of "short bursts" with small step-by-step increases in the rate that you burn oxygen and other key components of PACE, you get a winning combination. PACE is the only complete program designed to reignite your **native fitness**.

Reference: Jaret P. A Healthy Mix of Rest and Motion. *The New York Times*. May 3, 2007

Later I came to call this pattern the "Jim Fixx Phenomenon," after the popular fitness guru of the 1970s. Fixx claimed that the secret to heart health and long life was endurance running – up until he died of a heart attack – while running.

In the early 1980s, the same thing happened to Jack Kelly. Jack was the brother of actress Grace Kelly. He was also an Olympic oarsman and a president of the US Olympic Committee. He went out for his usual morning run and dropped dead of sudden heart failure.

This happens because adding repeated "cardio" to our busy days and pushing for greater endurance produces the **opposite** result of what we need in the modern world.

Unfortunately, the tragedy continues.

In 2006, at least 6 runners lost their lives in marathons in the US. In March, two police officers, one 53, the other 60, died of heart attacks at the Los Angeles Marathon. Three runners in their early 40s all had fatal heart attacks during marathons in Chicago, San Francisco and the Twin Cities. And on October 29th, at the Marine

Corps Marathon, a 56-year-old man collapsed at the 17th mile marker, never to recover.[3]

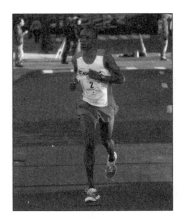

In 2007, two high-profile marathon related deaths occurred in the United States, one in Chicago and one during the Olympic trials in New York. A third runner died during the London marathon.[4]

In 2008 a young woman collapsed and died three miles from the finish line during the Dallas White Rock Marathon.[5] And at the New York City Marathon two men died during the race and a third runner died a week later. There was also a fatality at the Little Rock Marathon the same year.

These tragic deaths are not by chance. Marathon running puts an unnatural stress on your heart. And there's clinical evidence to prove it.

Science Finally "Discovers" the Risks of Marathon Running

Dr. Arthur Siegel, the director of internal medicine at McLean Hospital in Massachusetts and an assistant professor of medicine at Harvard University has authored more than two dozen studies on runners of the Boston Marathon.

In October of 2001, Dr. Siegel published two studies in the *American Journal of Cardiology*.[6] Between 1996 and 2001, he drew three blood samples from middle-aged male runners. He drew the first sample just before the marathon. He drew the second sample immediately following, and then a third sample a day after the marathon.

The results: 24 hours after the race, the men – none of whom had any history of heart disease – exhibited early-stage signs of cardiac damage strikingly similar to the symptoms that appear during a heart attack.

Results from Boston area hospitals reveal the risks and damaging effects experienced by dozens of marathon runners studied over the last ten years.

Increased Risks for Marathon Runners[7]	
• Heart Attack	• Sudden Cardiac Death
• Hardening of Arteries	• Stress Fractures
• Lower Back Pain	• Blood in Urine
• Repetitive-Stress Injuries	• Permanent Bone Damage

In a more recent study – published in the medical journal *Circulation* – Dr. Siegel and his colleagues from Massachusetts General Hospital tested 60 runners before and after the 2004 and 2005 Boston Marathons. Each runner had a cardiogram to look for abnormalities in heart rhythm.[8]

They also checked for evidence of cardiac problems in runners' blood. They used troponin, a protein found in cardiac muscle cells, as a marker of cardiac damage. If the heart is traumatized, troponin shows up in the blood. Its presence is also used to determine whether heart damage was sustained during a heart attack.

The runners (41 men and 19 women) had normal cardiac function before the marathon, with no signs of troponin in their blood. Twenty minutes after finishing, 60 percent of the group had elevated troponin levels, and 40 percent had levels high enough to indicate the destruction of heart muscle cells. In addition, most had noticeable changes in their heart rhythms.

MSNBC Warns About the Dangers of Long-Distance Running:

Are You Running Yourself to Death?
Participating in a Marathon
Can Put Severe Stress on Your Body

This is the headline that reminded the world of Dr. Arthur Siegel's groundbreaking research into the dangers of long-distance running.

His studies were published in the American Heart Association's journal *Circulation*. Results were sobering. The *"inflammatory storm"* triggered by the stress of running a marathon creates all the symptoms of heart disease.

As Dr. Siegel puts it, *"Your body doesn't know whether you've run a marathon… or been hit by a truck."*

The impact of these studies is consistently glossed over by the media. But the message is clear: your body was not designed for running marathons.

PACE makes long, boring routines a thing of the past. PACE consists of short bouts of intensity followed by rest and recovery. Total exertion is never more than 20 minutes.

PACE gives you bigger muscles, a leaner body, and more energy than you know what to do with… and you bypass all the dangers of traditional exercise.

Reference: McGrath T. Are You Running Yourself to Death?
http://www.msnbc.msn.com/id/27460551/. Updated Nov. 1, 2008.

Dr. Siegel said, *"Their hearts appeared to have been stunned."*[9] Exactly! During long-duration exercise, your heart is under constant stress with no time to rest and recover. If it goes on for long enough, your heart is traumatized and your body reacts by triggering a wave of inflammation.

Inflammation can be a good thing. It's a natural response to damage and it starts the repair process. But if you do this recurrently and 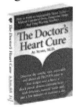 purposely as you exercise, you induce chronic inflammation of your heart and blood vessels – putting you on the fast track to heart disease. In *The Doctor's Heart Cure*, I showed that inflammation, NOT cholesterol, is actually the leading mechanism of heart disease.[10]

Dr. Siegel concluded that running a marathon causes injury to the skeletal muscles, which in his own words, *"sets off a cascade of inflammation in the body."* [11]

In yet another study, researchers at the University of Duisburg-Essen in Germany were surprised when men who had completed at least five marathons each were given an advanced type of heart screening called a spiral CT scan. This unique exam measures coronary artery calcification, or the amount of calcium plaque buildup in the arteries.

About 35 percent of the marathon runners had significant plaque buildup in their arteries, indicating they were at a higher risk for a heart attack. Only 22 percent of non-marathon runners in the control group had the same amount of blockage. *That's an increase in plaque buildup of over 50% in runners compared to non-runners.*[12]

New research led by Dr. Malissa J. Wood of the Cardiac Ultrasound Laboratory at Massachusetts General Hospital added a new layer to the picture of damage sustained by marathon runners.

Published in the November 2006 issue of *Circulation*, researchers used ultrasound and blood tests of 60 runners who finished the Boston Marathon. Test results showed some of the runners' hearts had trouble refilling chambers. Doctors also noticed abnormalities in how blood was pumped from the right side of the heart to the lungs.[13]

So why are studies finding these results?

Your Body Was Not Designed for Long-Duration Exercise

Routinely forcing your body to perform the same continuous cardiovascular challenge, by repeating the same movement, at the same rate, thousands of times over, without variation, without rest, is unnatural. This type of demand could have occurred rarely, but not in the daily environment of a native society in balance with its surroundings.

Yet nature has designed your body to adapt to whatever environment it encounters. Your body is not a simple machine. It's an adaptive organism that has its own intelligence – it is constantly adjusting how it rebuilds itself to try and stay in balance with its surroundings.

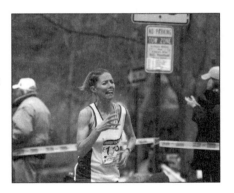

If you ask it to perform this activity repeatedly and routinely, it will gradually change the systems involved to meet the challenge more effectively. But what adaptive changes does this activity cause?

To help answer that question, think of your body as an engine with the additional feature of being able to gradually redesign itself.

If you want this engine to repeatedly go non-stop for long distances with low resistance, at a relatively slow speed, it will adapt to become more efficient at light, long, continuous, low output.

Long duration exercise produces some unique challenges your body must overcome. It must not run out of fuel, overheat or be overwhelmed with metabolic wastes.

One of the ways your body adapts is by gradually changing the capacity of your heart, lungs, blood vessels and muscles. To go those longer distances your body will give up maximal output while trying to keep the minimum "horsepower" required.

You wouldn't build a Formula-1 car to drive in a school zone. You'd waste fuel with a Ferrari sized engine going 20 miles per hour. And you'd waste money buying and maintaining a monster truck if you don't carry heavy loads.

Forced, continuous, endurance exercise induces your heart and lungs to "downsize" because smaller allows you to go further... more efficiently... with less rest... and less fuel.

Traditional Exercise Shrinks Your Heart's Output

So what's wrong with increasing durational capacity through downsizing? Instead of building heart strength, it robs your heart of vital *reserve capacity*.

Your heart's reserve capacity is that portion of its maximal output that you don't use during usual activity. To reuse the car analogy, your reserve capacity is the "pedal" that you have left on your accelerator before you hit the floorboard when you're cruising at your typical speed.

Think of it as money in the bank. If you have $50,000 in your checking account, you won't be bothered by a $1,500 repair you didn't expect. But if you live paycheck to paycheck and your credit cards are maxed out, any surprise could mean financial disaster.

Your heart works on the same principle. If your heart is in good shape and you only use 40 percent of its capacity during your normal daily routine, you'll have enough reserve power to help you when you need it. But if you don't have any reserve power, a sudden stressful event can trigger a heart attack.

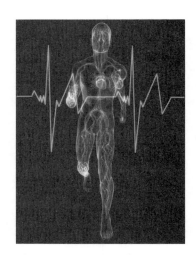

So if you downsize your heart and lungs you have traded greater reserve capacity for greater efficiency. This forces them to operate dangerously close to their maximal output when circumstances challenge them. For your heart, this is a problem you don't need.

Heart attacks don't occur because you lack endurance. They occur when there is a sudden increase in cardiac demand that exceeds your heart's capacity. Giving up your heart's reserve capacity to adapt to unnatural bouts of continuous prolonged duration only increases your risk of sudden cardiac death.

Dr. Siegel's research at McLean Hospital near Boston is not the only clinical evidence to reveal the dangers of durational exercise.

A groundbreaking study of long-distance runners showed that after a workout, the blood levels and oxidation of LDL (bad) cholesterol and triglycerides increased. They also found that prolonged running disrupted the balance of blood thinners and thickeners, elevating inflammatory factors and clotting levels – both signs of heart distress.[14]

That's bad news. You don't want LDL cholesterol to oxidize. Under normal conditions LDL cholesterol is your friend, not your enemy. But when small cracks and tears appear in the lining of your blood vessels it triggers inflammation. And inflammation causes LDL to oxidize and harden inside those cracks.

In simple terms, long-distance running activates the cycle of inflammation and LDL oxidation that causes artery-hardening plaque to clog your blood vessels.

CVE is bad for your bones too. A study published in the *Journal of Clinical Endocrinology & Metabolism* found that long-distance runners had reduced bone mass. This is true for both men and women – and women had an increased risk for osteoporosis as well.[15]

Long-Duration Exercisers
Showed Signs of Heart Distress
Increased LDL Cholesterol & Triglycerides
Shrinking Muscle Mass
Increased Oxidation of LDL Cholesterol
Elevated Clotting & Inflammation Factors
Loss of Bone Density and Increased Risk of Osteoporosis

These changes do not reflect a heart that's becoming stronger after exercise. And many of the subjects in this study stopped the exercise complaining of boredom.

Exercising for long periods makes your heart adept at handling a 60-minute jog, but it accomplishes this by giving up its ability to rapidly provide you with big bursts when circumstances might demand.

The real key to prevent heart disease and protect and strengthen your heart is to activate the opposite adaptive response produced by continuous cardio and *increase* your heart's reserve capacity. Bigger, faster cardiac output more immediately available on demand is what you really need.

Recent clinical studies show us the benefit of avoiding long-duration routines and exercising in shorter bursts.

Researchers from the University of Missouri found that short bouts of exercise were more effective for lowering fat and triglyceride levels in the blood.[16] (High triglycerides dramatically increase your risk of heart disease.)

Another study revealed the *duration* of exercise routines predicts the risk of heart disease in men. They found that several shorter sessions of physical activity were more effective for lowering the risk of coronary heart disease.[17]

The dangers of long-duration exercise are not limited to marathon runners. Even those free exercise classes at your local gym can cause problems.

Conventional wisdom tells us you need programs like "aerobics" to keep your heart in good shape. But as you'll see in the next chapter, this too is little more than a myth.

Endnotes

1 Lee IM, Sesso HD, Oguma Y, Paffenparger RS Jr. Relative intensity of physical activity and risk of coronary heart disease. *Circulation*. 2003;107(8):1110-11166.

2 Lee IM, Hsieh CC, Paffenparger RS Jr. Exercise intensity and longevity in men. The Harvard Alumni Health Study. *JAMA*. 1995;273(15):1179-1184.

3 Reynolds G. Is Marathoning Too Much of a Good Thing? *The New York Times*. Dec 7, 2006.

4 McGrath T. Are You Running Yourself to Death? http://www.msnbc.msn.com/id/27460551/. Updated Nov. 1, 2008.

5 McGraw D. Runner Collapses, Dies at White Rock Marathon. *The Dallas Morning News*. Dec. 15, 2008.

6 Siegel A, Stec JJ, Lipinska I, et al. Effect of Marathon Running on Inflammatory and Hemostatic Markers. *Amer Jour Card*. 2001;88(8):918-920.

7 Willdorf N. Run for Your Life?; *The Boston Phoenix*; http://www.bostonphoenix.com/boston/news_features/other_stories/multipage/documents/02229150.htm. Updated Apr 11, 2002.

8 Neilan TG, Januzzi JL, Lee-Lewandrowski E. et al. Myocardial Injury and Ventricular Dysfunction Related to Training Levels Among Nonelite Participants in the Boston Marathon. *Circulation*. 2006;114(22):2325-2333.

9 Ibid.

10 Sears A. *The Doctor's Heart Cure*. Dragon Door Publications, Inc; 2004

11 Ibid.

12 Möhlenkamp S, Lehmann N, Breuckmann F, et al. Running: the risk of coronary events: Prevalence and prognostic relevance of coronary atherosclerosis in marathon runners. *Eur Heart J*. 2008;29(15):1903-1910.

13 Neilan TG, Januzzi JL, Lee-Lewandrowski E. et al. Myocardial Injury and Ventricular Dysfunction Related to Training Levels Among Nonelite Participants in the Boston Marathon. *Circulation*. 2006;114(22):2325-2333.

14 Liu M, Bergholm R, Makimattila S, et al. A marathon run increases the susceptibility of LDL to oxidation in vitro and modifies plasma antioxidants. *Am J Physiol Endocrinol Metab*. 1999;276(6 pt 1): E1083-E1091.

15 Hetland ML, Haarbo J, Christiansen C. Low bone mass and high bone turnover in male long distance runners. *Journal of Clinical Endocrinology & Metabolism*. 1993;77(3):770-775.

16 Short bouts of exercise reduce fat in the bloodstream [press release]. *American College of Sports Medicine*. Aug 5, 2004.

17 Lee IM, Sesso HD, Paffenparger RS Jr. Physical activity and coronary heart disease risk in men: does the duration of exercise episodes predict risk? *Circulation*. 2000;102(9): 981-986.

PACE Success Stories:

"My family has a history of heart disease. So I decided I didn't want to be part of that particular bit of history. I decided to be proactive and sought out Dr. Sears' advice. About a year ago, I started PACE. I started out doing it 3 days a week. And in no time I started to see results.

I then started doing body-weight exercises to go along with PACE. One of the exercises I did was chin-ups. When I first started I could only do three.

I now do PACE for 20 minutes, 6 times a week along with my body-weight exercises 3 times a week. I am proud to say that I can now do three sets of 8 chin-ups!

In addition to my exercise I have been following a low-glycemic diet, eating foods with an index under 45.

I have lost 13 lbs. But what's more amazing is the fact that I am leaner than I have been in years. My body fat percentage went from 35% just one year ago to only 16% today.

I sleep better and I have so much energy. I feel amazing..."

Bob D., Naples, FL

&°~

"I use PACE for every workout and love my body more and more every day! I bought skinny jeans that didn't fit and now fit beautifully. In fact, I get so many comments from friends about how small my legs are getting! Yeah! Thank you!"

Sandi J., Henderson, NV

CHAPTER THREE

Aerobics Put to Rest

Remember Jane Fonda's workout video or Richard Simmons jumping around in spandex? Well, finally that exercise trend is dying. But not soon enough! "Aerobics" is not the way to exercise.

- It won't make you lean.
- It won't protect you from heart disease.
- It won't even boost your energy.

Even worse, aerobic training – the kind most doctors and even the federal government tout as the path to good health – can actually wreck your body. Do it for long enough, and aerobics will make you sick, tired and old before your time.

When you exercise aerobically, you have to keep the intensity at the medium level. If you increase or decrease the exertion level much, it is no longer aerobic activity. I'll explain this more later.

At this low rate, you have to work out for a long time before it will do anything. These repeated bouts of moderate intensity, long duration exertion are not as natural as you might think – and will likely cause you problems.

Let's get back to our car analogy. A small engine might be fine for long road trips. But if you need extra power fast, you're in trouble.

By staying in your "aerobic zone," you can never give your strength, power or capacity any challenge. This has the effect of shrinking your heart's output and restricting your lungs. This is the adaptive response your heart and lungs make so they can withstand long-duration workouts.

But as a result, you lose your reserve capacity – the ability to get extra power fast.

Think of this extra power as the "turbo" in your car. You don't need turbo power in normal traffic. But if you need to make a quick getaway, that turbo will get you out of trouble by giving you extra power at the moment you need it.

In your everyday life turbo power is essential. There are many activities that need extra oxygen and increased blood flow, like lifting something heavy, climbing stairs, jumping away from an oncoming car, or enjoying a night of lovemaking. These activities all require extra energy fast.

Sometimes an emotional shock needs the support of that extra power. It's common for people – especially elders – to suffer a heart attack after hearing terrible news about a loved one.

Reserve capacity means your heart and lungs have the power to get more oxygen to every cell in your body at a moment's notice.

It's easy to see why running requires more oxygen. Your cells burn through energy very quickly and need more oxygen to replenish their supply. But other events in your life require quick bursts of fresh blood and oxygen too.

That's why reserve capacity is critical. If you get hit with an unexpected expense and don't have money in the bank you'll wind up broke. If you get hit with an unexpected demand for oxygen and you don't have any reserve capacity you could wind up dead.

The real irony here is that our modern forms of exercise have taken away your reserve capacity. PACE is designed to give it back.

How did we get so far off track? Back in the late 1960s, Dr. Kenneth Cooper published *Aerobics* as the "perfect" way to "train" your heart and boost your aerobic conditioning. He thought that *medium intensity* aerobic exercise practiced three or four times a week was all you needed for health and longevity.

But this theory was never really proven. And there's plenty of evidence to support PACE style workouts. A recent study by Harvard researchers shows that those who do short-duration, high-intensity workouts reduce their risk of heart disease by **100 percent more** than those who practice aerobic

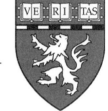

exercise.[1] Lead by researcher I-Min Lee, MBBS, ScD, the study came from the Department of Epidemiology, Harvard School of Public Health, Boston, Massachusetts.

What's more, *medium intensity* exercise does not build reserve capacity – or to refer back to your car – your turbo power. To do that, you need to kick it up a notch and do a higher intensity routine.

Skip Your Aerobics Class and Discover Your *Supra*-Aerobic Zone

A few years ago, a patient of mine – EP – came to me very out of shape. He said his cardiologist told him to never exceed his "aerobic threshold" when he exercised. Crossing the aerobic threshold means switching from medium intensity to high intensity. In the aerobics world that's a cardinal sin.

But here's the problem: If you never cross that threshold you never signal your body to increase lung strength and reserve capacity.

To better understand what your aerobic threshold is, we need to take a closer look at *metabolism*.

Metabolism is how the cells in your body process different nutrients to obtain energy. In your muscles, *adenosine triphosphate* (ATP) is the molecule they use for energy. Your cells have two different systems to generate ATP, *aerobic* and *anaerobic*.

ATP molecules are the basic unit of cellular energy. It's the first source of energy your muscles use. But you don't have a lot of ATP on hand at any given time. After a few seconds, you have to replace the ATP you burned if you want to continue the activity you're doing – whether it's walking, running, etc. The more you exert yourself, the more ATP your body needs to make.

Let's say you're walking down the street. At first, your body will use available ATP to feed your muscle cells. Then to replenish ATP, your body kicks in its *aerobic metabolism*.

Aerobic means "with oxygen." So your aerobic metabolism combines oxygen with carbs, fats and proteins to make ATP. Because walking is not a strenuous activity, you can easily obtain enough oxygen to make all the ATP you need. Using this model, you could walk for hours and not run out of fuel and not feel too tired.

But let's say you start jogging. The faster pace requires more energy. That means your cells will use oxygen more quickly. To keep the system working, you have to breathe harder to get more oxygen into your cells. At the same time, your heart starts to beat faster in order to get the oxygen to muscle cells more quickly.

Jogging is a typical aerobic exercise because it can be sustained with oxygen metabolism (aerobic metabolism). But what happens when you ask your body for more?

Let's say you start sprinting. For the first five or ten seconds, you can sustain that high output with oxygen – but not for much longer. After that five or ten second burst you can't produce ATP with oxygen fast enough. Pretty soon your muscle cells are depleted.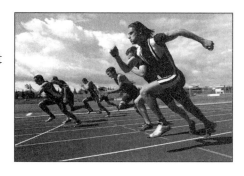

That's the point at which your *anaerobic* energy system kicks in. This is also known as crossing your **aerobic threshold**.

Anaerobic means "without oxygen." This system converts carbs – and some fats – into energy without using oxygen. This will sustain you in a sprint for a while. You can get a very high-energy output from this system but not for very long. And you'll notice that when you stop sprinting you will continue to pant heavily for oxygen.

Panting means that you've created an *oxygen debt*. This occurs when your muscles ask for more oxygen than your lungs can supply at that moment – like when you're sprinting.

Understanding when the anaerobic system kicks in is critical. When you're using your anaerobic system, you are training your high-energy output system. That's the "turbo power" that gives you extra power when you need it.

High-Intensity Exercise Best Way to Reduce Anxiety, University of Missouri Study Finds

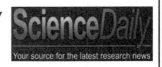

ScienceDaily (July 15, 2003) — COLUMBIA, Mo. – Cardiovascular disease is the leading cause of death in the United States. The amount of stress and anxiety a person experiences is a major factor in cardiovascular disease. For the past three decades experts have vacillated in their recommendations concerning the amount and intensity of exercise required to alleviate stress and anxiety.

Recently, most experts have agreed that a moderate to low amount of regular exercise can ease personal tension and stress. However, a new study by researchers at the University of Missouri-Columbia shows that a relatively high-intensity exercise is superior in reducing stress and anxiety that may lead to heart disease. Moreover, the researchers found that high-intensity exercise especially benefits women.

These results surprised researchers… but my patients who practice PACE tell me endless stories about the mental and emotional benefits of PACE.

Here's why: the high-intensity portion of my PACE program ramps up your levels of human growth hormone (HGH) and helps restore optimum brain chemistry. This has a direct impact on the way you think and feel. PACE reduces anxiety and supports a healthy feeling of optimism. I call it your "feel good factor."

But remember… the evidence supporting high-intensity training is just one piece of the puzzle. Combining all the elements of PACE gives you the complete strategy for native fitness. The mental and emotional benefits of high-intensity training are just a taste of better things to come.

Reference: *Science Daily.* Jul 15, 2003. Adapted from materials provided by University of Missouri-Columbia.

When this happens, you are successfully building up reserve capacity in your heart, expanding your lung volume, triggering the production of growth hormone and melting away fat.

For all these years, doctors, trainers and fitness "gurus" have been telling us to never cross that aerobic threshold – because they believed in the myth of aerobics.

But let's take this a step further… And this is a big misunderstanding I want to set straight: aerobic and anaerobic can only be used to describe *metabolism*. Like in the above description.

Aerobic and Anaerobic Don't Apply to Exercise

This is where modern exercise science has steered us in the wrong direction. It's possible for your cells to make energy without oxygen – but it's impossible for you to *exercise* without using oxygen. Therefore, there's no such thing as anaerobic exercise.

When you're sprinting, your body will start its anaerobic metabolism, but you are still breathing – still using oxygen. In fact, when your anaerobic system kicks in, your aerobic system is still functioning. *One does not replace the other.*

Aerobic energy production is simply limited in how much energy it can produce per unit of time. If you exceed that rate, you will continue to produce the maximum energy you are capable of with aerobic metabolism. But now you will add more energy from your anaerobic energy system.

So the term anaerobic exercise really makes no sense. I have a better term. When you've exceeded your aerobic limit and are exercising more intensely than aerobics, I call it **supra-aerobics**. You are exerting yourself at a higher than aerobic level but you are still using your aerobic energy systems as well.

By shedding this aerobics dogma and training yourself to find your **supra-aerobic zone**, you're going to restore native health benefits remarkably fast: A bulletproof heart, powerful lungs, strong muscles, youthful features, no excess fat and a long life.

A study published in the *Archives of Internal Medicine* showed that men and women who exercised with supra-aerobic methods had: [2]

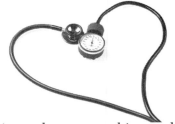

- Lower blood pressure
- Lower triglycerides (blood fat)
- Higher HDL (good cholesterol)
- Less body fat

Let's take a closer look at how aerobics and supra-aerobics stack up…

Aerobics	Supra-Aerobics
• Teaches your body to burn muscle mass	• Teaches your body to burn fat and build muscle
• Diminishes your lung capacity	• Increases your lung capacity
• Reduces your secondary sexual features. Men, you'll lose your broad shoulders and deep voice. Women, you'll lose breast tissue and your curvy figure	• Enhances secondary sexual features – builds a desirable, attractive figure
• High rate of injury	• Low rate of injury
• Lowers your overall energy levels	• Raises your energy levels
• Takes 60 to 90 minutes, 5 times a week	• Takes 12 to 20 minutes, 3 to 4 times a week
• Hard to stick with	• Easy to stick with

www.pacerevolution.com

Your Ancient Ancestors Used
Their "Supra-Aerobic Zone"

Until recent times – and until "experts" told us not to – we have always, at times, exerted ourselves with extreme intensity and purpose. All animals are either predator or prey. In the case of the human animal, we were both. We still have the genetic make-up to respond to the challenge – and we need to.

As my insightful colleague, Dr Phil Goscienski put it in his *Health Secrets of the Stone Age*:

"Most modern humans do not exercise as if their lives depended on it – but they do... If we don't push our heart and lungs toward their limits they will have little reserve, incapable of meeting the demands of stress, infection or injury."

"Thousands of generations ago (we) may have become another creature's meal... Now ...

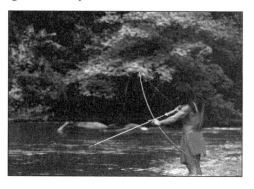

(we) are just as surely killed by diseases that were almost nonexistent, even in the elderly, back in prehistory. Instead of death that came in seconds, however grisly those last seconds must have been, our dying takes years." [3]

With short bursts of intense exercise, your body burns the energy stored in muscle tissue, instead of energy stored as fat. This teaches your body to store more energy in the muscles – not as fat – so it's available for quick bursts of energy.

The Daily Telegraph

Leading British Newspaper Reveals:

Six Minutes of Exercise a Week "Is As Good As Six Hours"

Just six minutes of intense exercise a week does as much to improve a person's fitness as a regimen of six hours, according to a study. Moderately healthy men and women could cut their workouts from two hours a day, three times a week, to just two minutes a day and still achieve the same results, claim medical researchers.

The two-minute workout requires cycling furiously on a stationary bike in four 30-second bursts. Professor Martin Gibala, the author of the study, said: "The whole excuse that 'I don't have enough time to exercise' is directly challenged by these findings. This has the potential to change the way we think about keeping fit."

This article shares the findings of a leading research team at McMaster University in Ontario, Canada and highlights one of the PACE principles: **short bursts of intensity**.

Later in the article, Dr. Gibala added:

"We thought there would be benefits but we did not expect them to be this obvious. It shows how effective short intense exercise can be."

This is no surprise… short bouts of high-intensity exertion trigger adaptive changes in your body. Blood sugar is used more efficiently, fat is easily burned and your performance ability skyrockets.

But intensity is only one part of PACE. To be effective – especially over time – applying rest, recovery and progressive changes are critical. These are the missing pieces most researchers overlook.

Reference: Zimonjic P. Six Minutes of Exercise a Week is as Good as Six Hours. *The Telegraph*. Jun 5, 2005

Aerobics Myth BUSTED!
Lactic Acid Is Not Your Enemy... *It's Fuel*

Finally, one of the last "old theories" of aerobic training is crumbling under the weight of new evidence. At the center of the breakthrough is *lactic acid*.

You've probably heard of it, especially if you've ever had a coach or a trainer. Conventional wisdom said you had to avoid lactic acid because the build-up in your muscles caused the pain, fatigue and soreness you feel after "overdoing it."

We were told to exercise aerobically and not cross the dreaded **lactic threshold**. Lactic acid starts to build in the muscles when your anaerobic system kicks in. The idea that you had to avoid lactic acid helped spur the aerobics craze that reached its peak in the 1980s.

But this theory never jived with the real world experience of the benefits of exceeding your aerobic threshold (which would build lots of the dreaded lactic acid). It turns out lactic acid is **not your enemy**. To the contrary, it's fuel for your muscles.

Dr. George Brooks from the University of California at Berkeley recently found that lactic acid is taken up and burned for energy by your mitochondria – the energy factories in your muscle cells.[4] What's more, it cannot create the after workout soreness because it is rapidly removed as you burn it for fuel. In other words, it's long gone before you get sore.

A short, intense, supra-aerobic workout is exactly what your body needs to increase your lungpower, build reserve capacity in your heart and melt away your fat stores.

Remember… aerobic exercise is low to medium output held for an extended period. Supra-aerobic exercise is high output, but short in duration. Why is this important? For one thing, it restores an element of your native environment.

Our ancestors lived in a world where their food fought back. Predators attacked without notice. They had to run or fight – fast and hard. These short bursts of high-output activity fine tuned our ancient ancestors and kept them fit. We still have the same physiology yet have lost that kind of challenge.

To move your workout into the anaerobic range, the key feature is this: Create an "oxygen debt" as I described earlier. Simply exercise at a pace you can't sustain for more than a short period. Ask your lungs for more oxygen than they can provide.

The difference between the oxygen you need and the oxygen you get is your oxygen debt. This will cause you to pant and continue to breathe hard even after you've stopped the exertion until you replace the oxygen you're lacking.

Here's another example: let's say you pedal as fast as you can on a bike for 15 seconds. When you stop, you continue to pant. This is the kind of high-output challenge you can't sustain for very long. You have reached your *supra-aerobic zone*. This is very different from doing an aerobic workout for 45 minutes.

This is the basis for your PACE program. I began using most of this program 25 years ago. More recently, I added *progressivity* to increase the benefits.

By making small changes in the same direction, your workouts can produce remarkable results. And you only need 12 minutes to achieve the desired effect.

In a matter of weeks, you can:

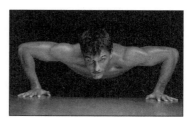

- Build functional new muscle
- Reverse heart disease
- Build energy reserves available on demand
- Strengthen your immune system
- Reverse many of the changes of aging

But hasn't modern exercise science proven that cardio and aerobics are the best way to get rid of body fat?

Actually, it's also a poor tool for getting lean...

Endnotes

1 Lee IM, Sesso HD, Oguma Y, Paffenbarger RS Jr. Relative intensity of physical activity and risk of cardiovascular disease. *Circulation* 2003;107 (8): 1110-1116.

2 Williams P. Relationships of heart disease risk factors to exercise quantity and intensity. *Arch Intern Med.* 1998;158(3):237-245.

3 Groscienski P., *Health Secrets of the Stone Age.* 2nd ed. Oceanside, CA:Better Life Publishers; 2005.

4 Kolata G. Lactic Acid is Not Muscle's Foe, It's Fuel. *The New York Times.* May 16, 2006.

PATIENT STORY

Joel and Carolyn Senter – Cincinnati, Ohio
From an email sent to Dr. Sears' office on January 29, 2009:

"You have probably heard on the news about the weather up here in the north. We have had ice and snow, lots of both. Today, my husband and I thought that we should try to start to dig out. My husband is in his late 70s and I am in my middle 60s. Both would be considered senior citizens. BUT, we've been doing PACE and eating the way Dr. Sears says and taking his nutrients for about 3 years.

Today I 'stepped off' the area of our driveway and it is almost 1000 square feet. It was covered in ice, which ranged from 3/4 inch to almost 2 inches. On top of the ice was about 4 to 5 inches of snow.

So, there we were chopping, shoveling, and thanking Dr. Sears because the only reason we stopped to take a break was because my husband's toes were too cold.

We still have plenty more to chop and shovel since we have about 1″ or more of ice and about 4″ of snow on top. I just wanted to tell you that we are drawing on that reserve that Dr. Sears talks about, but that reserve is there because we have been doing what he says.

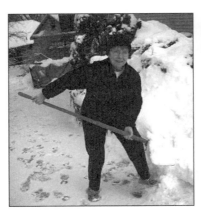 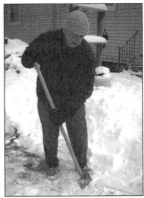

Later, we came in, took hot showers, had dinner and marveled at how we didn't hurt or ache or even feel unusually tired.

Please thank him for us. Tomorrow, we're off to chop and shovel some more."

Carolyn Senter

PACE Success Stories:

"I used to spend approximately 1.5-2 hours a day in the gym 5-6 times a week, BUT my weight never changed and I did not see any improvement. In the end, I was just exhausted. At one point I was even gaining weight. I thought that there is something wrong with my health.

I started PACE only recently. I have been doing it for about 2 months now and I ABSOLUTELY LOVE IT. I feel the same way as I felt after 2 hours of exercising… pleasantly tired, sweating like a pig and having tension in my muscles that gives me this sense that I did something for my body.

Now I have more time for myself, instead of running home from the gym, taking a shower, grabbing some lunch and out of the door to work. Now I can sing in the shower, slowly enjoy my lunch and I still have time left before I head to work."

Marina T., New Canaan, CT

છ્જ

"I am 6' 4", 260 lbs. but I have been unable to shed unwanted fat pounds even though I would do 1 hour on the elliptical. With PACE I now do 15 minutes on either the elliptical, treadmill or swim sprints. I love it mostly because it has shortened my workout by 45-50 minutes while making me feel better.

One more thing, I love to sing and after my first day with PACE, I could sing with more power while holding a longer note. I love it."

Frank M., Las Vegas, NV

CHAPTER FOUR

Relight Your Native Afterburner

Burn More Fat by *Avoiding* Your Fat-Burning Zone

Many in the exercise industry will tell you "cardio" and aerobics are essential for you to burn fat and get lean. They tell you to get into your "fat burning zone," and stay there for as long as possible. Yet there are several problems with this exercise theory.

For starters, consider the experience of body builders. Many of the very leanest people in this sport (some of the leanest people on the planet in fact) insist that part of their success was because they never do cardio.

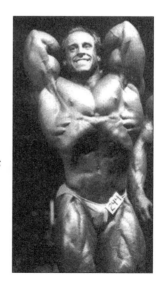

As a good example, John Defendis, former Mr. USA and world-class bodybuilder, told me he, "*never does cardio.*" He, like many others in his field, feels that avoiding cardio is the only way to keep your muscle and stay lean.

In his own words, John says, "*The key is not to do cardio, because you'll lose muscle. The idea is to increase your lean muscle. To do that effectively you must intensify and be progressive with workouts. I tell everyone I train to <u>never do cardio</u>.*"

I don't recommend body building, but when someone 280 pounds with the incredibly low body fat of 4% reports that he got that lean while *avoiding* cardio, it raises an interesting question about the necessity of cardio training to achieve low body fat percentages.

And, science gives bodybuilders more reasons to avoid cardio. A study published in the *Journal of Applied Physiology* shows the muscles of long-distance runners actually shrink.

When the muscle biopsies of 7 marathon runners were analyzed, researchers found their muscle fiber size had decreased and atrophied.[1]

Compare sprinters to marathon runners. Sprinters like Olympic gold medalist Carl Lewis – who use workouts similar to PACE – have lean, muscular bodies. Marathon runners on the other hand often have sunken chests and too much belly fat.

How about native hunters vs. native farmers? Hunters spend less energy in shorter bursts but have nearly universally lower body fat than farmers who spend hours of durational exertion in the fields all day. Many factors could account for this observation. But again, the association of shorter exertion with lower body fat raises a valid point.

Conventional wisdom asks us, "Don't you have to exercise for at least 15 or 20 minutes before you get into your fat burning zone?" After all, that's what the fitness gurus tell you. To answer that let's look at a simple model of our metabolism.

Your body can select from several fuel sources. It can burn fat, it can burn carbohydrates like glycogen or it can get energy from breaking down protein.

When you exercise for different lengths of time or different intensity levels you change the amount of energy you get from each of these three sources.

For the first couple of minutes, your body uses something called ATP – the most readily available source of energy. But your supplies of ATP are limited. After 2 to 3 minutes, your body switches to carbs stored in muscle tissue. This lasts for 15 to 20 minutes before you switch to fat.

As you'll see, this means your PACE routines are very short – never consisting of more than 15 to 20 minutes of total exertion.

But your body makes fuel choices based on your activity level as well.

Look at the table below.

What Does Your Body Use for Fuel?			
Activity Level	Protein	Carbs	Fat
Resting	1 to 5 %	35 %	60 %
Low Intensity	5 to 8 %	70%	15 %
Moderate Intensity	2 to 5 %	40%	55 %
High Intensity	2 %	95 %	3 %

Adapted from: McArdle W, Katch F, Katch V. *Sports & Exercise Nutrition*. New York, NY: Lippincott Williams & Wilkins;1999.

From the chart, you see that at low intensity activity your body derives most of its energy from carbohydrates and only 15% from fat. When you look at the lifestyle of our ancient ancestors, this makes sense. Low intensity activity – like walking long distances – was natural for hunter-gatherers.

Even today, long walks are effective exercise. And, as Henry David Thoreau once said, *"Walking is exercise for the soul."*

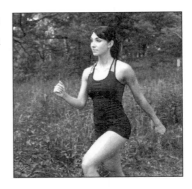

But when you step up your activity level to moderate, you increase the percentage of the energy burned from fat to 55% of the total. Notice that if you increase your activity to high intensity you dramatically reduce your dependency on fat and derive nearly all your energy from carbs.

These numbers inspired people to exercise at moderate intensity because that's how you burn the most fat. Although this seems logical, it turns out to be the wrong advice for getting lean.

To help explain, remember the analogy of your body as an engine but with the added feature of changing itself to better meet recurrent demands. What adaptive response do you induce by burning fat as your principle fuel?

Your body builds more fat to better prepare itself for medium-intensity activity.

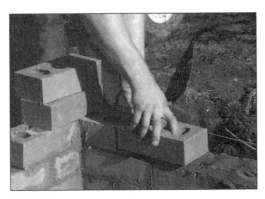

Here's another way to look at it: Imagine for a moment you're a bricklayer. Every morning you kneel down in your backyard and lay brick for two hours. One by one you stack them up with a layer of mortar in between.

What do you need to continue this hobby long term? A lot of bricks!

Now imagine your neighbor takes notice and delivers a new load of bricks to your house every morning. Being a helpful neighbor he wants you to have all the materials you need to practice your bricklaying.

> *"I have lost 17 pounds over 9 months. I have not changed my diet – I've used PACE. I love being in and out of the gym in such a short time."*
>
> David A., Sydney, Australia

This is the process your body goes through when you practice long-duration, medium-intensity exercise.

You need fat to burn when you exercise at medium intensity for long periods. Like the good neighbor who delivers a new load of bricks every morning, your body delivers a new layer of fat to provide you with the materials you need for long-duration exercise.

Are You Telling Your Body to Make More Fat?

Burning fat during exercise tells your body it needed the fat. *This trains your body to make more fat for the next time you exercise.*

Your body replenishes your fat each time you eat and becomes efficient at building and preserving fat necessary for long aerobic sessions in preparation for the next endurance workout. In doing so, it sacrifices muscle and preserves fat.

So don't bother trying to use this strategy to lose body fat. Your body will fight you in the effort and you can only do it by sacrificing lean tissue like muscle and internal organs.

And if the sole purpose of your exercise was to maximize energy derived from fat, why not just rest? Notice from the table that your body burns a higher percentage of fat (60%) *while resting*.

Think about it... you burn fat at a higher percentage of calories burned by watching TV than you do running on a treadmill! The fitness gurus who preach cardio because of the percentage of calories derived from fat seem to overlook this fact.

Durational exercise tells your body to build fat. That's how your body adapts to this kind of activity. Then, if you stop your cardio routine, you'll put on even more fat very rapidly. This is common as your body gets into the routine of making the extra fat.

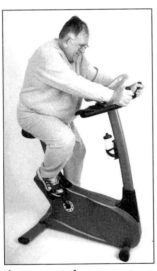

It's an endless cycle. And eventually, nearly everyone stops doing cardio. Most stop because they can't continue to devote the time because it takes so long. Many just get bored. Others find they have to stop cardio because this unnatural activity has caused degeneration of their joints.

And another point: If you persist with this unnatural exertion through middle age and beyond, cardio accelerates some very negative effects of aging. It doesn't just shrink your lungs; in my patients I've seen it lower testosterone and growth hormone, boost destructive cortisol levels, and rob you of muscle, bone, organ mass and strength.

But short-duration exercise – like PACE – actually *increases* levels of growth hormone. Researchers from Loughborough University in Leicestershire, England tested growth hormone levels in sprinters and endurance athletes. On average, the sprinters had 3 times as much growth hormone as the endurance runners.[2]

The biggest point they missed is this: The most important changes from exercise occur *after, not during*, the exercise period. The way you exercise affects your metabolism for several days. The important changes begin after you stop exercising.

This is good news. It means all you have to do during your exercise is stimulate the adaptive response you need – like reducing your need for fat or building reserve capacity in your heart. Your body will continue making the important changes afterwards – while you rest.

Burn Up to 9 Times MORE Fat by Exercising LESS

Short bursts of exercise tell your body that storing energy as fat is inefficient, since you never exercise long enough to use the fat during each session. Instead you burn carbohydrates, which are stored in muscle – not fat. Carbohydrates stored in muscle are high-energy output fuels while fat is a low energy output fuel.

Exercising for short intense bursts will use these high output carbs during exercise. Then you start to use slow-burn fat *after* your workout – while you replenish the carbs. This is known as your "after burn." And it, over the long run, is more important than what you burned during your exercise.

To illustrate just how powerful the effects of this afterburn are, take a look at this: Researchers in Quebec's Laval University divided exercisers into two groups: long duration and repeated short duration.[3] They had the long duration group cycle 45 minutes without interruption. The short duration group cycled in multiple short bursts of 15 to 90 seconds with rests in between.

The long duration group burned twice as many calories, so you would assume they would burn more fat. However, when the researchers recorded their body composition measurements, the interval group showed the most fat loss. In fact, the interval group lost *9 times more fat* than the endurance group for every calorie burned!

You may be thinking – doesn't this defy the laws of physics? Not really, when you realize that exercise continues to affect your metabolism after you stop. The short bursts stimulated a greater afterburn. In my practice, even I must admit to being surprised by the power of short bursts to burn fat and make people lean when cardio hadn't.

In addition, exertion in brief bursts will produce other benefits to your metabolic health that may surprise you. It will:

- Improve your maximal cardiac output.
- Promote quicker cardiac adjustments to changes in demand.
- Achieve "higher peak stroke volumes during overload." (Your peak stroke volume is the greatest amount of blood your heart can pump per beat when maximally challenged.)
- Improve your cholesterol profile. (People in a study of exercise bursts showed a decrease in total cholesterol and an increase in "good" cholesterol).[4]
- Provide a great anti-aging benefit by raising your testosterone, which fights against memory loss, accumulation of fat, low libido, sexual dysfunction, and loss of strength and bone.[5]
- Make you lose weight in less time by burning much more fat after you *stop* exercising.

And, you'll be able to get these benefits with much less of your time – no need to spend hours at the gym.

PACE: A Cure for Modern Times

Short Bursts of Exercise Proven More Effective Than Aerobics for Treating Metabolic Syndrome

Metabolic syndrome is a collection of symptoms that lead to chronic diseases like cancer, diabetes and heart disease. It's a common condition and rates are rising every year. Almost 25 percent of adults and 12 percent of children have metabolic syndrome.

This cluster of symptoms include:

- High blood pressure
- High blood sugar
- Abnormal cholesterol levels
- High insulin
- Excessive fat around the belly

Metabolic syndrome is one of the leading indicators of future disease.

In a new study published by the *American Heart Association* researchers discovered high-intensity exercise was hands down the best way to treat metabolic syndrome. It left aerobics in the dust.

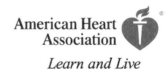

After just 16 weeks, almost 50 percent of the people practicing PACE-style movement were ***declared free of metabolic syndrome***.

PACE may be a cure for modern times.

(Continued on the next page…)

(Continued from the previous page...)

According to the study, *"high-intensity exercise is superior to moderate-intensity training in reversing the risk factors of the metabolic syndrome."*

Just look at the results. PACE-style training:

- Improved VO$_2$max (a measure of lung function and use of oxygen) twice as much as aerobic training.
- Boosted levels of NO (flexibility of blood vessels and sexual performance) while aerobic training showed no gains.
- Reduced oxidized LDL (bad cholesterol) by 17% while aerobic training showed no reduction.
- Showed a "significant improvement" in fasting blood sugar compared to aerobic training.
- Pumped up HDL (good cholesterol) by 25% while aerobic training showed no improvement.

Reference: Tjonna AE, Lee SJ, Rognmo O, et al.
Aerobic Interval Training Versus Continuous Moderate Intensity Exercise
as a Treatment for the Metabolic Syndrome: A Pilot Study.
Circulation 2008;118:346-354. Originally published online Jul 7, 2008.

Turn Up Your Body's "Fountain of Youth" Hormone

New research has uncovered startling changes that take place in your body within hours of starting PACE. (I've seen these same results in my own patients.)

Here are just a few of the added benefits:

- **Raise Your Levels of Human Growth Hormone (HGH):** HGH is your body's "anti-aging" hormone. It's been shown to build muscle, burn fat, improve bone density, raise your "good" cholesterol, and reverse the negative effects of aging.

Blood levels of HGH rise dramatically during and immediately after PACE-type exercise. (Traditional aerobic exercise has no effect on HGH.)

- **Burn More Calories:** PACE turbo-charges your metabolism. After intense bursts of exercise, your body needs to burn extra calories to repair muscles, replenish energy and bring your body back to its "normal" state. This process takes anywhere from a few hours up to a whole day – meaning you'll burn calories long after your workout is over.

- **Tap the Strength of Large Muscle Fibers:** Regular aerobic exercise uses smaller muscle fibers, as these fibers are more oxygen efficient. PACE draws upon larger muscle fibers, which generate more power but get tired more easily. Moderate aerobic workouts tend to ignore these larger fibers, leaving them weak and shrunken. By exercising these larger muscle fibers, you get stronger muscles that can handle heavy-duty demands. (Critical for mobility and independence as you get older.)

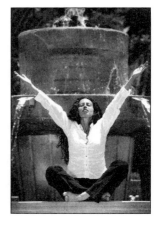

- **More Strength, Greater Fitness in Less Time:** After a few weeks of a "cardio" routine, you stop making progress and hit a "plateau." PACE helps you break through those dead spots and keeps you moving forward. Within just a few months of PACE, you'll be able to pump more blood and deliver more oxygen to your muscles – raising your energy levels like never before.

- **Bigger, Stronger Heart:** The PACE program gives your heart a boost you'll never get from traditional aerobic exercise.

Because PACE demands more oxygen, your heart adapts by increasing both its heart rate and stroke volume (the amount of blood your heart can pump in one beat). This increased pumping power makes your heart stronger – and last longer.

Burn MORE Fat While Saving You Precious Time

One thing you must do differently from previous standard exercise routines is to *decrease* the length of time for each exercise interval. As your conditioning increases, you will use shorter and shorter episodes of gradually increasing intensity.

For instance you may begin with 20 minutes every other day... then break those 20 minutes into smaller "mini-intervals" as you get into better shape.

> *"I need considerably less time to exercise and I feel fit, have more endurance, energy and can easily control my weight."*
> George P., Laranca, Cyprus

Shorter episodes will help you keep your muscle. When I taught anatomy and physiology classes at Barry University, I emphasized that muscles do more than facilitate movement. Your muscle mass is interconnected to your *metabolism* in the following ways:

- Fights fatigue, illness, sagging skin and bone fractures.
- Helps maintain a proper glucose balance.
- Increases your metabolic rate, reducing fat gain.
- Strengthens your immune system to decrease disease risk.
- Helps you to perform daily activities necessary for an independent quality lifestyle.
- Stores glycogen, which provides energy for the body.

This never-ending need for muscle continues throughout your

life, especially as you reach your 60s, 70s and beyond. People with greater muscle mass benefit from proficient mental functioning, fewer chronic illnesses and a longer, healthier life.

PACE helps you build new muscle and it puts your body into fat burning mode – *automatically!*

Mike Started PACE and Lost 97 Pounds of Fat...

Mike gave me permission to share his statistics and progress with you, as further proof of PACE results.

When Mike first visited me, he had 50% body fat and took 11 drugs for his physical problems. In just **12 weeks**, he lowered his body fat to 30% and in **18 months**, Mike achieved a body fat score of 10%.

As you can see from the chart below, Mike also lost 66 pounds from February 2002 to April 2003. What's more, he threw away the prescriptions for the 11 drugs he was taking.

Date	02-08-02	04-22-02	02-05-03	04-29-03
Weight	283	263	226	217
Skin Fold				
Chest	48	30	10	6
Abdomen	60	42	12	8
Thigh	50	30	20	14
TOTAL	158	102	42	28
% Body Fat	42%	31%	14.4%	10%
Pounds of Fat	119	82	33	22
Lean Body Mass	164	181	193	195

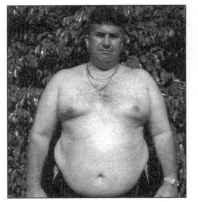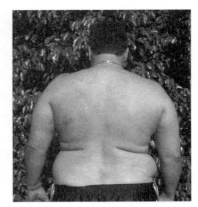

Mike - Before PACE

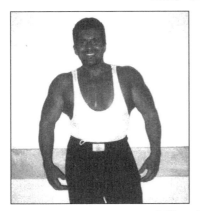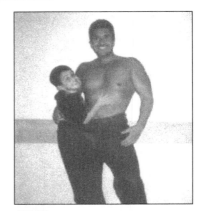

Mike - After PACE

Proof of PACE in Action: Dr. Sears' Twin Study

My **Wellness Research Foundation** put PACE to the test in a clinical study of two identical twins. When they arrived for their initial assessment, both twins – age 18 – had almost identical body composition measurements. (Body composition measures the amount of body fat and lean body mass, or muscle.)

At the start of the study, both twins ran one mile each, three times a week. Over the course of 16 weeks, the "PACE" twin progressively *decreased* her distance to fit the PACE program. The "cardio" twin progressively *increased* her distance to match a traditional cardio routine.

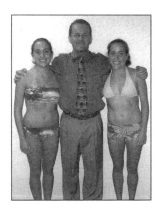

By the end of the study, the PACE twin was **sprinting** 6 exercise sets. Each set had a 50-yard exertion interval followed by a recovery period of 30 seconds. The cardio twin was **jogging** 10 miles straight with no breaks.

The results? The PACE twin went from 24.5% body fat all the way down to 10% for a total fat loss of 18 pounds. What's more, she gained 9 pounds of pure muscle.

The cardio twin lost fat, but not as much. She also started at 24.5% body fat but went down to only 19.5% body fat for a total fat loss of 8 pounds. Not bad, but instead of gaining valuable muscle, the cardio twin actually *lost* 2 pounds of muscle. Here's a look at their stats:

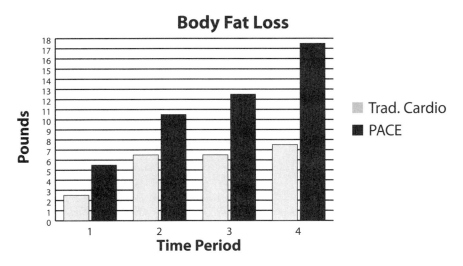

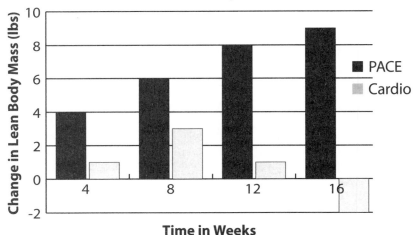

Lean Body Mass

Note that the PACE twin gained 9 pounds of muscle during the study period while the cardio twin lost muscle. But even more striking – **the PACE twin lost more than twice as much body fat** than the cardio twin. And she did it while exercising for one quarter as long.

And that's just the beginning. As you'll see later, some of my patients have experienced even more profound results. All using the same easy-to-follow principles you're learning right now.

Endnotes

1 Trappe S, Harber M, et al. Single muscle fiber adaptations with marathon training. *J Appl Physiol,* 101:721-727, 2006.

2 Vanhelder WP, Goode RC, Radomski MW. Effect of Anaerobic and Aerobic Exercise of Equal Duration and Work Expenditure on Plasma Growth Hormone Levels. *Eur J Appl Physiol* 1984;52(3):255-257.

3 Tremblay A, Simoneau JA, Bouchard C. Impact of exercise intensity on body fatness and skeletal muscle metabolism. *Metabolism.* 1994;43(7): 814-818.

4 Murphy M, Nevill A, Neville C, Biddle S, Hardman A. Accumulating brief walking for fitness, cardiovascular risk and psychological health. *Med Sci Sports Exerc*. 2002; 34(9): 1468-1474.

5 Kraemer WJ, Häkkinen K, Newton RU. Effects of heavy-resistance training on hormonal response patterns in younger vs. older men. *J Appl Physiol*. 1999:87(3) 982-992.

PATIENT STORY

Name: Byron Black
Age: 67
Diagnosis: Obesity and Diabetes
Home Town: Burleson, TX
From a letter sent to Dr. Sears' office:

"I saw Dr. Sears in December of 2007 wanting help with losing weight. My weight at the time was 250 lbs. I was on a number of different types of medications and I was taking four injections of insulin a day. Prior to my visit to Dr. Sears, I had blood tests done so he would have a baseline of where I was at that time.

The first thing we discussed was a new type of eating. He provided me with a Glycemic Index for most types of food. He instructed me not to eat anything on the list over 35.

Second, we discussed exercise and what I was doing at the time. He then told me about his PACE Program. He instructed me on how to start and build on the PACE Program to help all aspects of my health.

It has now been 9 months and my weight is between 210 and 215 pounds. I no longer take insulin injections, and I take only two prescriptions now. My resting heart rate is 45 to 50 when I get up in the morning and my blood pressure continues to be at a normal level.

The comparison to when I had my first visit with Dr. Sears is one of having my life back. One that is full of energy and with no highs or lows. A freedom that comes with insulin no longer poisoning my body and taking away years from my life. I am no longer a prisoner of poison that was depriving me of life. I have been able to finally lose the weight I have so desperately wanted for several years. Each day I have felt better and that has made it easy to stay with the diet.

My family has noticed a change in me. They remark on the added energy, and the ability to enjoy life free from insulin. They say they have their Dad back like he was when he was younger. My wife notices the changes each day. She supported me during the years of diabetes and has supported me in this new phase of my life. She sees a happier, healthier person who is not dying before her eyes."

Byron Black

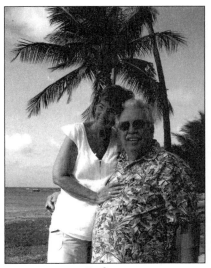 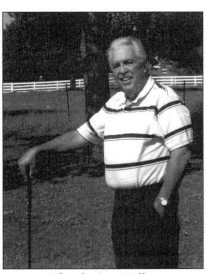

Before   **After losing 40 lbs.**

CHAPTER FIVE

Join the PACE Revolution Now

After seeing the flawed conventional exercise theories exposed to logic and science, I hope you will now allow PACE to liberate the native fitness within you.

PACE is indeed a revolution. And it's growing...

Thousands of people from around the world practice PACE. And by the end of this chapter, you'll have in hand all you need to start PACE without difficulty, stress, or strain.

This chapter is completely self-contained. Even if you don't read any further, you'll have all the basic building blocks to get you started and keep you going.

Throw Off Decades of Misleading Exercise Advice... PACE Puts You on the Fast Track to Lasting Fitness

PACE is a complete and natural approach to fitness. Instead of forcing you into an artificial fixed routine, PACE simply leads you back to your own *native fitness*.

Your native fitness comes with the feeling of being effortlessly energetic with a naturally lean, high-performance body. It's the state of vitality that arises when your body is matched with, and in balance with, your native environment.

In ancient times native fitness was a given. It happened without effort. Our ancestors were physically challenged in ways that promoted lean muscle, strong hearts and robust lungs. And they faced these challenges *everyday*.

Over millions of years our human bodies developed, evolved and adapted along these lines. The body you have today is a result of this long-running, continuous fine-tuning. Genetically you are still identical to those ancestral hunters. But our environment has markedly changed.

Today we spend most of our time indoors. A "strenuous" day might mean lifting a box or carrying groceries. Gone are the days when we had to forage, climb, swim, hunt for our food or run away from predators to save our hides.

> *"Fantastic results – stronger, more cardiovascular fitness, gained 8 lbs. of muscle, lost 1/2 inch in waist, and not working out for hours on repetitive exercises. I love PACE."*
>
> Jerry N., Hillsborough, CA

And there's the rub.

Because we were built by that ancestral environment to match that ancestral environment, our bodies still need to be pushed in the same ways. Our physiological limits need to be explored, used and challenged. We don't get this from our current environment but the requirements remain. Challenge our maximal capacity or face living weak, fat, tired, crippled and diseased.

Challenging your maximum capacity requires the intensity of your exertion to "flirt," at least a little, with your current capacity...

but your capacity will change quickly when you challenge it… so your experience of intensity changes over time.

This is the most important element of the solution, of how to build back your native fitness: You only have to challenge your cardiopulmonary capacity a little bit at a time and your body responds with added heart, lung and skeletal muscle capacity while you rest. Then the next exertion period will feel easier because of your bigger lungs and stronger heart – so you PACE at just a little higher rate without really feeling an increase in perceived effort.

It never feels like a burden. PACE is enjoyable. You'll feel energized afterwards, not bored and exhausted. Just the opposite of what you may have experienced with aerobics and cardio.

PACE = *Progressively Accelerating Cardiopulmonary Exertion*®

Here's a quick overview of what PACE means:

The last two words in the acronym PACE are cardiopulmonary exertion. With this phrase I simply mean to give your heart and lungs a bit of a stimulus to do more – to provide more oxygen. You can use any physical activity that gets you breathing harder and increases your heart rate.

Now let's look at the two principles that make PACE unique and so remarkably flexible and effective.

Progressivity: Repeated Changes in the Same Direction

By progressive I mean repeated changes in the same direction. Exercise can dramatically change your body over time only when you change what you are doing over time. You have to do a little more of one component each time you do it.

During your workout you will progressively increase the intensity of your challenge. There are many ways to do this. You will find a simple way in this chapter.

To have progressivity you have to change your routine over time. Doing the same routine over and over – especially with cardio and weight training – will lead to some minor gains at first but then your progress will stall. It's the usual reason for the fitness "plateau." Your body needs a new challenge in order to adapt and grow.

As you get more familiar with making progressive changes to your routine, they will become intuitive. Each time you do PACE strive to do something new, or a little more or somehow differently. These progressive changes will allow your body to continue to make adaptive responses, today and years into the future. Like interest on a bank account these little adaptive changes and little new challenges, can have a monumental cumulative effect.

Acceleration: Training Your Body to Adapt Faster to Demands

As you train your adaptive response, you will give it new demands a little faster as your body gets used to it. This will train your body to respond more quickly – and adapt more quickly – to the demands you make on it. As you train your body to respond faster each time you exercise, your physical condition improves faster as well.

This is the principle of acceleration.

When you start PACE, it will take several minutes to get your heart rate and breathing up. This is perfectly okay to still benefit when you are out of shape, or de-conditioned. But as you progress, you'll reach your target heart rate more quickly and your breathing will get deeper and more efficient sooner when challenged.

The same applies during your recovery. When you're out of shape it takes a long time to recover from exertion. But as you adapt, your recovery time shortens. Your heart rate comes down faster. Your breathing returns to normal more quickly. This too, is acceleration. These two features of the accelerating nature of PACE, with practice, have the added advantage that you don't need to increase the time you spend with PACE as you become more fit. In fact, I usually decrease total time because patients become quicker at both gearing up and recovering.

> *"The gift of this book is that it is the perfect marriage of modern science, medicine and practical fitness theory. Where else can one get the insights of a medical doctor who also knows his way around a workout room, track or swimming pool?"*
>
> Greta Blackburn
> Editor, M. Fitness Magazine
> Founder, FITCAMPS

You will be stimulating, encouraging and training the speed of the response time of your heart, lungs, blood vessels and metabolic machinery. So you train your physiology to have higher levels of fuel, oxygen and energy for you more immediately available on demand. This also has the priceless benefit of making you feel more energetic.

PACE Gives You the Space and Freedom to Be an Individual

Don't worry if you're not in "peak condition." With PACE you can start anywhere. Whether you're an amateur athlete or a stay-at-home mom, you can start PACE right away. You'll begin at a level that's comfortable for you.

PACE is flexible. You can do it anywhere, any time, with nothing more than a few spare minutes and a bit of space.

You can do PACE using any kind of machine or exercise you like. Of course, you can use your local gym to do your PACE program. But you don't *need* a gym, weights, or special machines. Your backyard will do just fine. Or a box or a flight of stairs or even a chair. Or the grassy hill at your local park.

You can even do PACE in your living room – and get exactly the same benefit as you would in a state-of-the-art athletic facility.

You won't struggle with the obstacles you may have faced with other fitness programs, either. You won't have to dedicate months or years of effort without anything to show for it. Your heart and lungs will respond immediately.

The results will come in a matter of weeks – sometimes in a matter of days. You'll start building muscle, shedding fat, and creating lifelong health and power from your very first workout.

And your first workout will take just minutes.

Getting Started: Your First PACE Workout

Your first PACE workout will be a single period of exertion followed by recovery. You will start at a speed and level of intensity that feels comfortable to you. Then you will gradually increase your level of intensity until you are panting and breathing heavily. When you reach this level of exertion you will stop and recover. That's it.

During your first workout you will make a few observations:

- How long does it take before you start breathing heavily?
- How long does it take for your breath to recover after you stop?
- What was your approximate heart rate during exertion?

This is the foundation of PACE. You start off easy, you gradually increase the intensity, you reach a level of maximum exertion, and you stop and rest.

As you progress you will have the freedom to improvise and make changes to your routine. But for now, these are the basics.

To get started, you can walk, run, swim or choose an "instrument." An instrument is simply an exercise device like a treadmill, a rowing machine, an elliptical, a bicycle, etc.

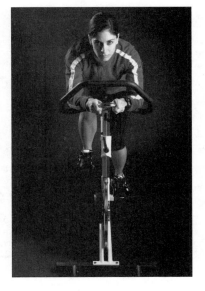

If you are out of shape or not sure how you will react when you exert yourself then you might consider walking. It will be easier to control your speed and is a safe place to start.

For now, let's say you're using a stationary bike.

Start by adjusting the seat and getting comfortable. The seat should be high enough to give you some leverage and pedaling power, but not so high that your legs become fully extended.

Set the resistance level to a low setting. You should feel a little tension but should be able to pedal freely and easily. Make note of the time. Start pedaling.

As you continue, start thinking about *perceived exertion*. This is how tired you *feel*. This is not a scientific measurement and will be different for everyone. But it's an important observation.

Use caution and always check with your doctor before starting this or any exercise program. Especially if any of the following factors apply to you:

Risk Factors

- Over 50 Years Old
- No Medical Checkup Within Two Years
- 25+ Pounds Overweight
- High Blood Pressure
- Heart Attack, Rapid Heart Palpitations, Chest Pain After Exercise
- Taking Heart Medication
- Angina, Fibrillation, Tachycardia, Abnormal EKG, Heart Murmur, Rheumatic Heart Disease
- Blood Relative Died From Heart Attack Before Age 60
- Asthma, Emphysema, or Another Lung Condition

Note: When beginning an exercise program, it's important to start out light and increase your effort over time.

Some of my patients feel a high level of exertion after walking for 60 seconds. Others can sprint for 50 yards and not even break a sweat. These are extremes at either end of the scale. For now, simply make note of how you feel.

After a few minutes of pedaling at low resistance, turn up the intensity. Pedal for another minute and turn up the resistance again. Keep pedaling. How quickly you turn up the resistance is up to you. But here's the idea: **Progressively increase the intensity over time.**

If you're feeling out of shape, do it slowly. If you have more experience, you can jump into a more intense level earlier on. As you keep pedaling, your level of perceived exertion will increase. You'll start to sweat. Your face will feel flush. Your breathing will get faster and deeper.

Keep turning up the intensity until you've reached your limit. How do you know when you've reached this point? Simply stated, you'll run out of steam. You'll start to pant. Your breathing will be uncontrollably heavy.

When you're in this state you won't be able to speak clearly. Your breathing will be too deep and demanding.

At this stage you've created an oxygen debt. This occurs when you ask your lungs for more oxygen than they can give you in that moment. That's why your breathing quickens and deepens. Your body is trying to get as much oxygen as quickly as it can.

Now rest. Stop pedaling.

Make note of the time. How long did it take you to get winded? One minute? Ten minutes? It doesn't really matter. There's no right or wrong answer. This is your *exertion time*. It's your baseline, your starting point.

> "PACE has indeed helped me. I have better lung capacity. My strength and endurance have increased. I feel better, stronger. I've lost half off my excess waist measurement and I look better."
>
> Martin H., Colorado Springs, CO

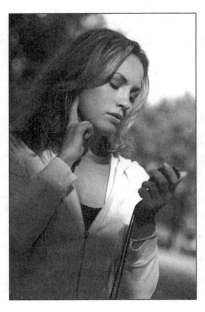

Now reach up and take your pulse. The easiest place to find your pulse is on your neck. Feel around the area of your wind pipe. When you're winded and breathing heavily you'll feel a robust and vigorous pulse. Look at your watch and count your pulse for six seconds. Now multiply by ten. That's your **heart rate**.

For example, if you find your pulse and count 14 beats in six seconds your heart rate is 140. (14 x 10 = 140)

Now relax. Make note of the time. You want to see how long it takes you to "get back to normal" after you finish. It might take you 4 minutes… it might take you 20 minutes. This is your **recovery time**. Again, you are simply observing and taking notes.

How do you know when you're back to normal? It's about *perceived recovery*. This is not a scientific measurement. It's when you *feel* rested. It's when you feel like you've "caught your breath."

Now take your pulse again. Write it down.

That's your first PACE session.

Let's review. During your first exertion period followed by recovery, you:

- Chose your instrument and started at a comfortable, low-intensity level.

- Progressively increased the intensity.
- Continued until you felt a high level of exertion.
- Created an oxygen debt while breathing heavily.
- Stopped and rested.
- Made note of your heart rate and exertion and recovery times.

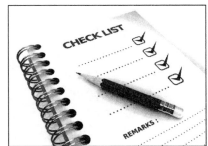

There are many different ways to do PACE. You only need to use its principles. But your PACE will always follow this basic structure: You alternate between exertion and recovery, while making progressive changes.

Now that you have the hang of it, let's give your PACE program a little more structure. This will help you practice PACE on a regular basis.

Below you have three basic examples of PACE.

Each one has a different feel.

You can take these workouts to the gym, to the park or stay in the comfort of your own home. You can use any instrument you like. Again, it's your choice. If you feel like taking it slow, start by walking. If you're ready to experiment, try running up a hill or get into the gym and try using stair master.

Even better, you can cycle between these three workouts for as long as you like. Do each one for 4 to 6 weeks before trying the next. After you finish the third, go back and do the first, but change some element of the workout to make it different.

Ideally, you will practice PACE three times a week. But even if you can only manage one you'll be ahead of the game. PACE workouts are never wasted. The benefits start rolling in, even if you only do a single set.

> *"I finished reading PACE recently. I did my first 10-minute program this morning using Hindu squat for exertion and an exaggerated walk for recovery. I can feel it in the back of my thighs this evening! I'm excited about this!"*
>
> Richard N., Dover, MA

As with everything in life, consistency counts. You will make some gains from doing PACE once a week – or even once a month. But to get the body you really want... to maximize your true potential, I recommend three times a week.

This chapter gives you the basics of PACE, but you can stay with the basic program for as long as you need.

Once you're ready, you can take PACE to the next level. You'll find everything you need in the following chapters.

For now, let's have a look at the 3 basic PACE workouts.

Basic PACE Workout 1

Warm-Up	Set 1		Set 2	
	Exertion	**Recovery**	**Exertion**	**Recovery**
2 min	4 min	X min	3 min	X min

Set 3		Set 4	
Exertion	**Recovery**	**Exertion**	**Recovery**
2 min	X min	1 min	Done

Total exertion time: 10 minutes.

This workout features a descending pattern of exertion time as you progress through each set. For example, your first exertion period is 4 minutes. Your second is 3 minutes, etc.

As you begin each set you will increase the intensity. Your first exertion period is 4 minutes but your intensity level will be low. Your 4th set is only 1 minute but your intensity level should be high. You want to give this last set everything you have.

The recovery time is intentionally left open. Take as long as you need. But as soon as you catch your breath, start your next set.

Like all three of these basic PACE programs, you can apply any instrument or setting. You can do them indoors or out. You can do them walking, running, swimming, jumping rope, or do them in the gym. Any machine you like.

Basic PACE Workout 2

Warm-Up	Set 1		Set 2	
	Exertion	Recovery	Exertion	Recovery
2 min	2 min	X min	2 min	X min

Set 3		Set 4	
Exertion	Recovery	Exertion	Recovery
2 min	X min	2 min	X min

Set 5		Set 6	
Exertion	Recovery	Exertion	Recovery
2 min	X min	2 min	Done

Total exertion time: 12 minutes.

Instead of using a descending pattern with increasing intensity, this workout gives you 6 sets of 2 minutes each. This pattern is useful if you're outside running or going up a hill. But you can use instruments in the gym as well.

You won't be able to increase the intensity as much with this routine. Getting through 6 sets will challenge you all on its own. But start with a medium to medium-high intensity right from the start.

Slightly increase the intensity with each set.

By the time you get to sets 5 and 6 you will really have to push yourself to finish. You may fight fatigue, so if you have to slow down a bit that's okay. As you progress your performance will improve.

Basic PACE Workout 3

| Warm-Up | Set 1 | | Set 2 | |
	Exertion	Recovery	Exertion	Recovery
2 min	45 sec	X min	90 sec	X min

| Set 3 | | Set 4 | |
Exertion	Recovery	Exertion	Recovery
2 min	X min	4 min	X min

Total exertion time: 8 minutes, 15 seconds.

This PACE program is the opposite of the first program. Instead of starting with longer exertion periods and steadily decreasing, you'll start with a short, high-intensity exertion period and move on to longer exertion periods.

As you increase the exertion time of each set you'll slightly decrease the intensity. You may think this is easier... but this is just as challenging if not more so.

When you get to your last set, don't let the intensity drop. Keep it up. Push to the end.

You'll notice there's a lot of flexibility in these workouts. They're designed to give enough structure to practice regularly but enough freedom to give you room to grow.

The idea here is getting started. You can alternate between these three workouts for as long as you like. But get creative. Apply the element of progressivity. Change it up.

When you need to add something new to your routine here are a few ideas:

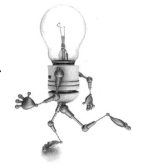

- Increase the pace of each exertion period.
- Add one more set to your routine.
- Add more resistance to each exertion period.
- Change your instrument.

Don't forget to keep track of your progress. Make note of your heart rate and your recovery rate.

As you progress, your cardiac output and your recovery time will improve. You'll notice your heart rate will climb higher and reach its target faster. And your recovery time will shorten. These are milestones you don't want to miss.

I'll give you more tips for tracking your progress in later chapters. First, I want to share a story with you. You'll learn a lot from Terri... her story starts at the end of this chapter.

PACE Gets Results FAST – Even If You're Out of Shape or Think You Can't Exercise

Many times my patients tell me they *want* to exercise and feel better… they just can't get around the roadblocks that get in the way.

These blocks can be physical, mental or emotional – or a combination of all three. It's very common to feel afraid or intimidated by physical exertion. And just as common to have an injury or health problem that makes you feel like exercise is impossible.

Even more typical is the frustration that comes from not seeing results. That may be the biggest stumbling block to staying fit.

> "I love [PACE]! I have lost considerable body fat and couldn't be happier! To think I could lose belly fat exercising 20 minutes was a dream that is now MY reality! I couldn't be more pleased."
>
> Danna G., Scottsdale, AZ

PACE is the antidote.

PACE is a "can do" activity regardless of how out of shape you are… or how discouraged or disabled you might feel.

Unlike aerobics, cardio or interval training, PACE lets you start anywhere – and make small, progressive changes that get you in shape regardless of where you started. *And you see results quickly.*

Case Study: Terri Lyttle
Age: 56
Source: Ongoing research through Dr. Sears' clinic and Wellness Research Foundation

When Terri first came to my office she weighed 250 pounds and told me she felt like she was *"dragging her feet all the time."*

Even daily chores drained her energy. When Terri went to her local mall the extra walking would trigger lower back pain and leave her fatigued. When she went to the beach, she would feel exhausted just from carrying her beach chair a quarter mile from the parking lot to the shoreline. When she got out of the car or off the couch she would strain and hold her breath as she rallied to get up.

In terms of exercise, Terri said she had tried everything. During her first visit she ran down a list of routines and diets she had tried: pilates classes, gym memberships, cycling, swimming, fast walking, colon cleansing, weight-loss supplements, high-carb diets, low-carb diets, cabbage soup diets... *all with no results.* And each time she tried something and it didn't work out for her, she quit.

Her journey was typical of so many: a lot of starts and stops with nothing to show for it.

When she enrolled in the PACE program we did a round of blood work and measured her body composition. Because Terri agreed to a long-term study, I brought in one of my PACE-certified trainers, coach Scott Wood.

Coach Scott was one of the first fitness trainers to finish my PACE certification program. I trained him here at my clinic in

South Florida. He works with my patients and answers questions on my online PACE forum.

The program we designed for Terri is a great example of how you can start from nothing and completely change your level of fitness in a way that is non-threatening and easy to follow.

It shocks most people but Terri started doing PACE *by walking for 45 seconds, then stopping to rest.* It's true. All she did was walk for a few seconds and rest for a few seconds, then repeat. That was the level she felt comfortable with. It wasn't intimidating. In her words, *"It wasn't scary."*

Starting with a very humble and easy workout we slowly made progressive changes to each of Terri's workouts. Within the space of just a few weeks, Terri went from walking for 45 seconds to "power-walking" up steep hills. Today she can run, sprint and workout with weights. As you can see, Terri made remarkable progress:

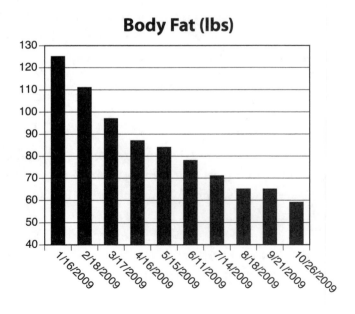

Body Fat (lbs)

www.pacerevolution.com

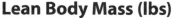

Lean Body Mass (lbs)

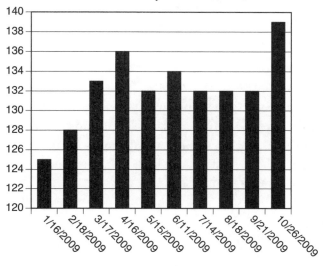

HDL (mg/dL)

Triglycerides (mg/dL)

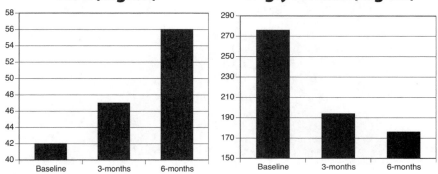

Over the course of nine months, Terri:

- Lost 66 pounds of fat
- Built 14 pounds of new muscle
- Raised HDL (good cholesterol) by over 30%
- Lowered Triglycerides (blood fat) by over 35%

PACE is proving effective across the board, from fat loss to cardiovascular health and beyond. Lowering triglycerides is especially helpful for Terri as triglycerides are more of a risk factor for cardiovascular disease in women than in men.

Terri's lungpower is on the rise, too.

Terri's office is on the second floor. Before she started PACE she would always take the elevator. Now she bounds up the 25 steps three or four times a day without thinking about it.

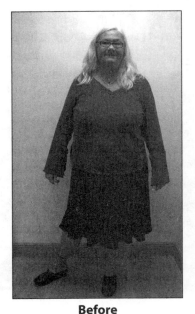 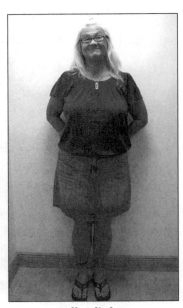

Before　　　　　　　　　　**66 lbs. lighter**

In Terri's own words, she describes PACE as, "*just so doable...*"

CHAPTER SIX

Unleash Native Fitness in 12 Minutes

When I introduce PACE to a new patient I occasionally hear the comment, *"Isn't PACE just a form of interval training?"*

I don't blame them for making the comparison.

Interval training – sometimes referred to as high-intensity interval training (HIIT) – shares a common feature of PACE. Both use short bursts of exertion followed by rest and recovery.

But that's where the similarities end. ***PACE is not interval training.***

Interval training *can* produce great results. Interval training techniques are used by professionals around the world to enhance their training programs and their track records.

But that's one of the problems with interval training: you need to be in great shape before you can use it effectively.

Most Olympic gold medalists and professional athletes regardless of their sport use interval training because it works. They seldom practice aerobics. And they don't run marathons unless that is their sport. They know better.

Carl Lewis is a good example. He's won more gold medals than any athlete in history. He endorses interval training and says, "*interval training has been used for decades by the world's greatest athletes.*"[1]

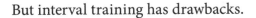

There's no doubt that interval training works. There are hundreds of clinical studies showing the effectiveness of short, high-intensity workouts. I'll share some of them with you in this chapter.

But interval training has drawbacks.

Interval training was originally designed for elite athletes who could train at a very high level. For the non-athlete you must be in excellent physical condition before you can even attempt the routines. After all, not everyone can do 8 sets of sprints at 100 yards each without any practice or prior training. (Some of my patients can barely walk.)

PACE allows you to start from any level of conditioning. If you can stand up, you can do PACE. It has a progressive element that helps you achieve a competent level of fitness regardless of where you started. Remember Terri from the last chapter? She started out walking for just 45 seconds. That's a far cry from the heavy demands of interval training.

Keep in mind that interval training tends to be a fixed routine – just like aerobics and cardio. The supporters of interval training may disagree. But everyone I talk to who uses interval training falls into the same trap: They don't change their workout. They may use short bursts of high intensity, but they do the same thing over and over.

When your body gets used to a particular routine it stops adapting. As a result you hit a dead spot in your training. This is often called a *plateau*. A plateau is a barrier that prevents you from making progress. It's very common in cardio and aerobics. But it happens with interval training too.

As you've read in earlier chapters, PACE works because it continues to create an *adaptive response* with each new progressive change in PACE. It's the change your body makes after you give it a particular challenge that has the powerful cumulative effect.

You can create any type of adaptive response you want... good or bad. Exercise works. But what kind of adaptive response should you be training?

As bad examples, when you practice aerobics and cardio your body adaptively responds by decreasing your lung capacity and cardiac output. That's not the kind of response you want for long-term good health.

> *"With PACE, I'm able to exercise without pain or injury – which at my age, 70, is a good thing. I've also been able to increase the intensity of my workout. Compared to other types of cardio, I feel great."*
>
> Bill P., Brunswick, ME

Interval training will help your body increase its lung capacity and expand its cardiac output. That comes from using short bursts of high-intensity exertion followed by rest. But without the progressive element you hit a plateau. Your body stops responding. The benefits stop.

PACE overcomes the limitations of interval training by allowing anyone to get started, and by always changing some aspect of the workout.

PACE progressively increases the level of your challenge. By making small changes in the same direction you give your body the ability to adaptively respond over time. You never hit plateaus. You always progress.

PACE ensures a lean body, a healthy heart and a robust set of lungs. Exactly what you need to avoid disease and stay looking and feeling young.

Interval Training Is Not Really New… In Fact, It's Much Older Than the Aerobics and Cardio Crazes

Long before Jane Fonda started jumping around in her leg warmers, world-class athletes were using interval training to improve their performance times.

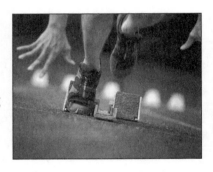

Interval training was formalized back in the late 1930's when German coach Woldemar Gerschler teamed up with Dr. Hans Reindell. Together they created the first interval training program: multiple sets of 200-meter sprints with intervals of rest in between.

They called it "interval" training because each burst of exertion was followed by rest. To them it was the most valuable part of the workout. They understood it was during the rest period that the bodies of their athletes made *adaptive responses*, i.e. – bigger lungs and stronger cardiac output.

According to their original workout, runners had 90 seconds of recovery. During that time they had to get their heart rate down to

120 beats per minute. If they needed more than 90 seconds it was an indication the workout was too difficult and needed adjustment.

Did they get results? You bet. The athletes they trained broke world records.

On July 15, 1939, Rudolf Harbig ran the 800-meter in 1:46.6 – beating the world record by a remarkable 1.6 seconds. This is still considered one of track and field's landmark performances. Less than a month later, Harbig set a world record for the 400-meter, finishing in 46.0 seconds.

Rudolf Harbig's 800-meter world record lasted 16 years until Roger Moens – another student of Coach Gerschler – finished in 1:45.7 in 1955.

Perhaps the most famous athlete to set a world record using interval training was Roger Bannister. In 1954, after incorporating the techniques of interval training into his daily one-hour training program he became the first man in history to run a mile in under four minutes.

The history of interval training and the clinical evidence that backs up its effectiveness is an important milestone in the history of fitness. It's the first time we've adopted exertion levels that mirrored our ancient ancestors. It's a step in the right direction.

But interval training has limitations. And it was never designed with **native fitness** in mind. It's just not practical for most people.

Imagine trying Coach Gerschler's workout… sprinting for 200 meters with only 90 seconds of rest in between. If you're out of shape this would be impossible. You might as well try and fly to the moon.

If you're not a professional athlete it takes more time to recover between exertion periods. *A lot more.* I had a patient who walked for just 30 seconds and needed 15 minutes to get her heart rate down. This is an extreme example, but not uncommon.

In our society we've stopped training for recovery.

This is a deadly mistake. Your heart and lungs were not designed for continuous exertion. You need dynamic rest. That's when your body makes important changes.

Unlike any exercise program that's come before it, PACE enables you to get fit, and stay fit, regardless of where you started. And it gives your body the chance to make the changes you need to stay lean, trim and disease free.

"I am so grateful to Dr. Sears and his creation of the PACE Program. As a busy mother of three small children, a wife and CEO, I simply do not have the time or inclination to spend working out unnecessarily. With PACE, just 12 minutes a day gives me the peace of mind that I am improving my mental and physical health.

In the second edition of PACE, Dr. Sears shares not only what to do but why to do it. And in a way that any non-medical person can understand and execute for fast results. In a recent exam and lung test in my doctor's office, he told me I have the lungs of a 30-year-old and I'm 48! After that I went home and got my husband started on the program as well. Now we have more time for each other and our kids!"

MaryEllen Tribby, Founder/CEO, WorkingMomsOnly.com;
Special Consultant to Early to Rise

Japanese Researcher Reveals the Science Behind Interval Training

During the 1990s, Dr. Izumi Tabata made sports science history at the National Institute of Health and Nutrition in Tokyo, Japan. Inspired by the interval training program used by Japanese speed skaters, Dr. Tabata initiated a now famous set of interval training studies. His most famous shows the powerful effects that short, high-intensity workouts have on your lungs.

He measured the VO_2max (the amount of oxygen that gets transported to cells in a given amount of time), and the anaerobic capacity of two groups of cyclists. One group did medium-intensity long-duration routines like aerobics for 60 minutes. The other did short, high-intensity routines like PACE for just 4 minutes.

After six weeks, the group doing the short, high-intensity workouts improved their VO_2max by 14 percent and their anaerobic capacity by a remarkable 28 percent.[2]

The high-intensity workouts not only improved their lung volume, but also raised the amount of oxygen their body could produce during their workouts. This performance boost enabled them to hit their supra-aerobic zone and trigger the adaptive responses that create a lean, disease-free body.

Dr. Tabata's program helped with fat burning too. The cyclists who did the 4-minute workout burned more calories in a 24-hour period than the cyclists who labored for an entire hour. In today's busy world it's easy to see the advantage of having a 4-minute workout.

As a result of his research Dr. Tabata developed what's often referred to as "The Tabata Protocol." This workout, based on his experiments became the new benchmark for interval training. It consists of 8 sets of 20-second high-intensity intervals followed by 10-second intervals of rest.

Gym-goers and athletes alike use the Tabata Protocol as their primary form of interval training. It's applied to all types of exercise including squats, pull-ups, push-ups, sit-ups, rowing and weight lifting.

Like other forms of interval training the Tabata Protocol can be effective when executed well. But it still has the same limitations. Its level of difficulty is very high and it's certainly not for everyone.

> *"After 30 days, I have lost 5 lbs. and 1 inch from my waist. I am 70 years old and I have noticed more energy and lung capacity. Great program. You are on to something BIG with this program."*
>
> Gerald P., Marysville, WA

The real value of interval training is what it teaches us: Short bursts of high-intensity exertion followed by recovery is the most effective form of exercise. It mimics the daily routine of our ancient ancestors and promotes native fitness.

The key is execution. If you have a coach or a skilled trainer, interval training may be a possibility. But most people don't. PACE on the other hand is accessible to everyone. No matter how overweight or out of shape you may feel, PACE makes real change possible.

The history of interval training gives us a valuable perspective on fitness. It's well researched and is backed up by decades of published, peer-reviewed clinical studies.

Aside from Dr. Tabata's published research, there are literally hundreds of others. To give you an idea I've included a few examples here.

Just 6 Sessions of Interval Training
Boosts Oxygen and Endurance

Researchers from McMaster University in Canada found just six interval workouts (short sprints) over two weeks increased oxygen available to muscles and doubled the runners' endurance capacity.[3]

High-Intensity Interval Training
Ramps Up Fat Burning in Only 2 Weeks

Another McMaster University study found that just seven sessions of interval training over two weeks marked a significant increase in fat burning for women.[4]

Interval Training Builds Muscle Function
and Improves Blood Pressure in Diabetics

Sports medicine scientists from the Netherlands used interval-training techniques with type 2 diabetes patients. In just 10 weeks diabetics showed better muscle function, lower blood sugar and lower blood pressure.[5]

Interval Training Strengthens the Lining of Blood Vessels

The lining of your blood vessels releases nitric oxide, which allows blood vessels to relax and dilate. This is critical for cardiovascular and sexual health. Researchers at the University of Missouri discovered that interval sprint training enhances the health and performance of the *endothelium*, the lining of your blood vessels.[6]

Professional Cyclists Resist Fatigue and Ride Faster

At the University of Cape Town in South Africa, cyclists improved their 40-km time trial performance and increased their muscular resistance to fatigue – just from a simple four-week interval training routine.[7]

Interval Training Better Than Aerobics for Your Heart and Lungs

When VO_2max (how much oxygen you can take into your lungs) and stroke volume of the heart (how much blood your heart pumps in one beat) were measured, interval training easily outperformed aerobics. VO_2max and stroke volume improved significantly more for people who used interval training.[8]

Case Closed: High Intensity Beats Aerobics and Cardio Hands Down

So the best way to fitness is high-intensity interval training (HIIT). But the question is how? The answer is PACE. PACE allows you to start anywhere and get to a level of fitness where you can do HIIT.

The studies above are just the tip of the iceberg. Interval training has a long history and plenty of clinical proof to back it up. But interval training is just one piece of the puzzle. The goal is *native fitness*. That's the state of vitality that arises when your body is perfectly matched to your environment.

PACE uses a facet of interval training but is designed to do much more. PACE reconnects you with the strength, power and natural muscularity your ancient ancestors enjoyed. That's your birthright.

What's more, PACE reconnects you with your natural instincts. Instead of plugging yourself into a fixed routine or something theoretical, PACE gets your blood racing. It sets you on fire. It gives you the exhilaration and intensity you could never get from jogging on a city street.

> *"I've only been on the program for a week, but I am very impressed by it. I can already see a difference in my heart rate recovery time, my resting heart rate and my energy level."*
>
> Joan W., Northampton, MA

PACE is an approach to exercise, not a set routine or theory like aerobics, cardio or interval training. PACE is fluid and adapts to your changing life. And by progressively adding new challenges, PACE lifts you up and puts you on the path of healing.

Endnotes

1 Nitti JT. *Interval Training for Fitness.* London: A&C Black Publishers; 2002.

2 Tabata I, Nishimura K, Kauzaki M, et al. Effects of moderate-intensity endurance and high-intensity intermittent training on anaerobic capacity and VO2max. *Med Sci Sports Exerc.* 1996;28(10):1327-1330.

3 Burgomaster K, Hughes SC, Heigenhauser GJ, Bradwell SN, Gibala MJ. Six sessions of sprint interval training increases muscle oxidative potential and cycle endurance capacity. *J Appl Physiol.* 2005; 98(6):1985-1990.

4 Talanian JL, Galloway SD, Heigenhauser GJ, Bonen A, Spriet LL. Two weeks of high-intensity interval training increases the capacity for fat oxidation during exercise in women. *J Appl Physiol.* 2007; 102(4):1439-1447.

5 Praet SF, Jonkers RA, Schep G, Stehouwer CD, Kuipers H, Keizer HA, van Loon LJ.. Type 2 diabetes patients respond well to interval training. *European Journal of Endocrinology.* 2008;158(2):163-172.

6 Laughlin MH, Woodman CR, Schrage WG, Gute D, Price EM. Interval training enhances endothelial function in some arteries. *J Appl Physiol.* 2004; 96(1):233-244.

7 Lindsay F, Hawley JA, Myburgh KH, Schomer HH, Noakes TD, Dennis SC. Improved athletic performance in highly trained cyclists after interval training. *Medicine & Science in Sports & Exercise.* 1996;28(11):1427-1434.

8 Helgerud J, Helgerud J, Høydal K, Wang E, et al. Aerobic high-intensity intervals improve VO2max more than moderate training. *Medicine & Science in Sports & Exercise.* 2007;39(4):665-671.

PATIENT STORY

Valerie

Valerie was the winner of my PACE Fat-Loss Challenge in 2008. She's a courageous and focused lady who is still losing fat and building her confidence, even though the challenge is over.

At one point, Valerie lost 13 pounds in one week. Overall, she used PACE to lose 40 pounds in six months, including 6 inches off her waist.

After her victory, Valerie said the best feeling was, "*being free of the food addiction I've had for so long...*"

Congratulations, Valerie. Job well done.

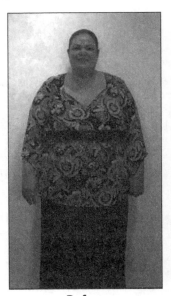 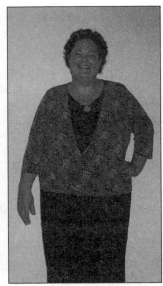

Before   **40 pounds lighter**

CHAPTER SEVEN

Track Your PACE Fitness

Getting on your bathroom scale every morning to see if you've made "progress" won't help you. It's not an accurate way to measure fitness.

When patients come to my office I measure their ***body composition***. That tells me exactly how much fat they're carrying… and how much lean body mass.

I also keep track of their heart rate and recovery time, and measure several features of breathing capacity. These measurements are a much better gauge of health and fitness. *And I recommend you keep track at home.* This chapter will show you how.

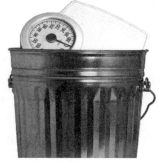

Heart rate and body composition are easy. To test your lungs, talk to your doctor about taking a *pulmonary function test*. You can also track your lung strength at home with a *peak flow meter*. They are designed for people with asthma, but you can use it as a way to monitor your lung strength between pulmonary function tests. Peak flow meters are small, portable and inexpensive. You can find them online.

Let's start by measuring your body composition.

Ignore "Experts" and Find Out If You're Fit or Fat

Measuring your body composition is a simple matter. But most doctors and fitness "experts" never bother. They rely on BMI or Body Mass Index. However, you need to know that BMI is an unreliable and outdated system. It's a calculation based on height and weight. *But it doesn't differentiate fat from muscle.*

Muscle is denser than fat and it will increase your BMI score more than fat will. That means having a lot of muscle will give you a high BMI, even if you are lean and trim. And this failure leaves BMI open to a *huge potential for error.*

> "*I have been getting fantastic results [with PACE] – lost 15 lbs. in one and a half months, down one pant size, and have gained inches in my arms and chest.*"
>
> Paul S., RN, Philadelphia, PA

My own BMI calculates to 29. This would lead you to believe that I'm overweight, almost obese. Yet, I have only 12% body fat.

Under the BMI system, people with a lot of muscle will have a higher score and will be considered "overweight" (BMI score of 25 to 29.9) or "obese," (BMI score of 30 or above) even though they may be extremely fit.

According to the BMI, these celebrities are "overweight":

Celebrity	Height	Weight	BMI Score
Michael Jordon	6' 6"	216	25
Will Smith	6' 2"	210	27
George Clooney	5' 11"	211	29

I bet these Hollywood insiders never realized they were "obese":

Celebrity	Height	Weight	BMI Score
Mel Gibson	5′ 9″	214	32
Arnold Schwarzenegger	6′ 2″	257	33
Sylvester Stallone	5′ 9″	228	34

Body composition measures how much of your weight is fat and how much is lean muscle mass. Men should have 10 to 20% body fat and women should have 15 to 25%.

There is little point in measuring more than once every two weeks. Once a month is usually enough for most people.

As you progress with PACE aim to increase lean body mass and reduce body fat.

The ratio of fat to lean body mass is your *real* measurement of health. To go back to our twin study from Chapter 4, here's the body composition of the "PACE" twin who lost 18 pounds of fat and gained 9 pounds of muscle over 16 weeks.

Date	Apr 7	Apr 28	May 19	June 2	Aug 18
Weight	118	116	113	113	109
% of Body Fat	24.5	19.5	16.3	14.2	10
Lbs. of Fat	29	23	18	16	11
Lbs. of Lean Body Mass	89	93	95	97	98

Notice her percentage of body fat dropped from 24.5 percent all the way down to 10 percent. By the end of her PACE program she had the body of a professional athlete.

You can easily measure your body composition at home:

1. **Electrical Impedance** – This is not the most accurate testing method (calipers are better), but it's easy. One version is a scale, similar to your bathroom scale at home. You enter a few numbers like your age, weight, etc. and it gives your body fat percentage.

   Another version is a hand-held device that looks similar to a video game controller. Like the scale you enter a few numbers then hold it with both hands. After a few seconds your body fat percentage appears on the screen.

   This method uses your body's conductivity to calculate your body fat, since water-based tissues are good electrical conductors and fats are insulators. You can find both types on the Internet.

2. **Skin Fold Test** – This is the most accurate and easiest way to measure your body composition. Using skin calipers, you measure skin folds to determine your percentage of body fat. In less than 5 minutes, you can get a correct measurement. You can find calipers on my website: www.alsearsmd.com.

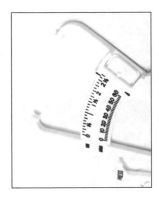

Your Heart Rate: The Key to Effective Exercise

Your pulse rate or heart rate is the speedometer of your heart. It tells you the number of times your heart beats per minute.

You can measure your heart rate at two pulse points: inside your wrist and the carotid artery in your neck. (The carotid artery carries blood to your brain and can be found by running your index and middle fingers along your windpipe.)

You will use three measurements to approximate your heart health and track your PACE progress:

- Resting Heart Rate
- Maximum Heart Rate During Exertion
- Recovery Time

Your pulse or heart rate is measured in beats per minute (bpm). Each "beat" is actually a contraction as your heart squeezes to pump blood. Your heart rate rises to meet the demands of an activity and then recovers when you rest.

Generally speaking, the lower your resting heart rate, the fitter you are – unless you have a pacemaker or heart disease.

The speed of your heart when you're at rest is your *resting heart rate*. As you start to exercise, your heart rate speeds up.

The "top speed" your heart achieves at the peak of your exercise routine is your *maximum heart rate during exertion*. This number will vary depending on your age and level of fitness.

People who are young or very fit can achieve a heart rate of 190 to 220 during exertion. On the other end of the scale, maximum heart rate might be 110 to 130. This is common if you're out of shape or recovering from surgery or heart disease.

The time it takes for your pulse to go from its exercise rate down to its resting rate is called your *recovery time*.

As you get into better shape your resting heart rate and recovery time will *decrease*. And your maximum heart rate during exertion will *increase*.

This is how you measure your heart's progress.

When you begin your PACE program don't be overly concerned or discouraged by your measurements. It's normal to have a high recovery time when you're starting out. Simply observe and take notes. You'll see steady improvements over time.

These three measurements are the key to making progress. However, many of my patients ask me about another measurement: "maximum heart rate." They say things like, *"Dr. Sears... my doctor told me never to go above my maximum heart rate for my age."*

This is a common concern. But as you'll find, guidelines designed for large groups of people are just that – *guidelines*.

> *"My legs look the way they did when I was in my 20s. They are firm, muscled and very strong. My arms are muscled and growing firmer every week. Belly is strong and flat. I feel better than I have – maybe ever.*
>
> *I've been health conscious since my 20s, but, in retrospect, I realize I never felt 100% good. Aches and pains are gone, my mind feels clear, and I feel happy every day.*
>
> *Did I say that I turned 69 this summer? When I hit 70, I will be in the best shape of my life. Thanks to your dedication to rectifying all the misinformation about diet, exercise and supplementation, I'm on the right track."*
>
> Linda C., Dallas, TX

Does Maximum Heart Rate Matter?

Your **maximum heart rate** is the highest number of times your heart can contract in one minute.

Textbooks and conventional wisdom calculate your maximum heart rate using your age. But is your maximum heart rate a useful number? Should you use it during exercise?

The answer is both yes and no. Finding your max heart rate based on your age is a good signpost. It's a reference. *But your PACE program is not fixed around this point.*

Your maximum heart rate actually achieved during exertion is more helpful.

Your maximum heart rate based on your age is a reference that's the same for everyone. If you're 64 years old your maximum heart rate is commonly defined as 156 bpm. That reference is true for everyone who happens to be 64 years old.

But it may not be true for you.

If you're 64 years old and very out of shape, 156 may be unrealistic. Your max heart rate may be lower. But after using your PACE program your max heart rate will likely increase. So any guide you use to gauge your heart rate should be flexible.

In the real world, rigid references are not always accurate. Let's look at how maximum heart rate is usually defined.

The most popular equation for figuring out maximum heart rate is **220 minus your age**.

According to this formula, if you're 24, your maximum heart rate is 196 bpm. (220 – 24 = 196) If you're 64, it's 156 bpm. (220 – 64 = 156)

This formula is still used and is the most common. But there is some controversy. Many feel it's not accurate.

The problem with the "220-minus-your-age" formula is that it slightly *overestimates* the maximum heart rate for younger people, and slightly *underestimates* the maximum heart rate for older people.

For a better estimate, this formula is more exact:

208 – [Your Age Multiplied By 0.7] = Maximum Heart Rate

If you're 60, multiply your age by 0.7. That gives you 42. Then subtract 42 from 208. That gives you 166.

Now that you've established this reference, what does maximum heart rate mean? How should it apply to your PACE routine?

Your maximum heart rate is simply a *guideline* for measuring your heart's level of conditioning.

If your max heart rate is "officially" 166 for your age (if you're 60), that doesn't necessarily mean you have to get your own heart rate that high. By the same token your max heart rate may be higher than 166. It depends on your level of fitness.

Gauge yourself as an individual. *An individual who is always in a state of growth and progress.*

PACE reflects life in motion. It's "progressive," not fixed or rigid.

Your max heart rate may be lower when you start your PACE program. Two years later, for example, your cardiac output may have increased dramatically giving you a new max heart rate.

Observing your current level, recording it, and comparing it to future observations will give you an ongoing measure of health. Use it as a tool. Not as an absolute.

The same can be said for the common advice, *"workout at 60 to 80 percent of your maximum heart rate."* You'll hear this from personal trainers. The idea is to get you into your "fat burning zone" during cardio or aerobics.

As you discovered in Chapter 4, you'll burn more fat by staying *out* of your fat burning zone. Keep in mind, working out at 60 to 80 percent of your max heart rate was designed for long-duration activities.

When you're doing your PACE program the "60 to 80 percent rule" doesn't apply. The primary goal is giving yourself a worthy challenge and progressively changing some aspect of your workout.

"I have been using PACE with my recumbent bicycle for about 8 weeks now. So far I have lost about 6 pounds and my clothes are looser. I am particularly grateful to PACE as I had spent months exercising with 'traditional aerobics' only to see no results or a few pounds of gain (ugh!). Finally, I feel like I have broken out of that rut and have momentum going toward weight loss and improved health."

Patty S., Newfane, VT

If you've pushed your limits and achieved an oxygen debt you've had a successful PACE workout.

If you want to monitor your heart rate and find some reference point that's fine. If you know you're getting your heart up to

70 percent of its maximum, that will act as a guidepost for you. A month or two later, you might find you're hitting 80 percent.

There's a big difference between exercising at 60 to 80 percent of your maximum heart rate and using it as a reference point. Forget the former and stick to the latter.

Here's a table with some max heart rates based on age. You'll also see how the numbers stack up when you calculate 60 and 80 percent of maximum.

Your Heart Rate Guide			
Age	Maximum Heart Rate (bpm)	60% of Maximum (bpm)	80% of Maximum (bpm)
40	180	108	144
50	173	104	138
60	166	100	133
70	159	95	127
80	152	91	122

Now that you're familiar with some of the terms, let's explore them further. This will help you find and use these critical measurements.

Find Your Resting Heart Rate

The average resting heart rate for an adult is between 60 and 100 beats per minute. Well-conditioned athletes can have a resting heart rate between 40 and 60 beats per minute.

To find your resting heart rate, do the following:

- Sit quietly for two minutes and then find your pulse.
- Count the number of beats you feel in 6 seconds.

- Multiply by 10 and write it down.
- Repeat this process two more times and record your results.
- Calculate the average of these three results.
- **This is your Resting Heart Rate.**

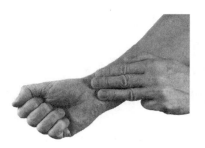

Number of beats in 6 seconds (1st time) × 10 = __61__

Number of beats in 6 seconds (2nd time) × 10 = __57__

Number of beats in 6 seconds (3rd time) × 10 = __61__

Total Beats ÷ 3 = _____60_____ **Resting Heart Rate**

(60)

Taking the measurement three times is simply a way to get a reliable average. Keep in mind that your resting heart rate will be a little higher if you've just had a cup of coffee or other caffeinated drink.

As you become more conditioned your resting heart rate will gradually become lower.

What Is Your Maximum Heart Rate During Exertion?

Your **maximum heart rate achieved during exertion** is the heart rate you achieve during your workout. It will change slightly from day to day.

This measurement is a more accurate gauge of your overall capacity. When you're first starting out, it might be lower than the max heart rate recommended for your age. But that's okay.

Here's an example: Let's say you're 60 years old. Your recommended maximum heart rate is 166 bpm. But during your workout you only get your heart rate up to 140 bpm. In that case your maximum heart rate during exertion is lower than the maximum heart rate recommended for your age.

So what do you do?

Using the actual results you get during a workout is always more useful. If all you can achieve is 140 bpm that's quite all right. That's your baseline, your starting point. It reflects you as an individual.

As your heart becomes stronger and your cardiac output rises, your maximum heart rate during exertion will increase.

Measuring is easy. When you're at the end of your exertion period – when you are winded and panting – record your heart rate.

You can do this a number of ways. If you're wearing a heart rate monitor simply make note of what it says within a few seconds of finishing your exertion period. If you don't have a heart rate monitor find your pulse on your neck and look at your watch. Count the number of beats you feel for six seconds and then multiply by ten. So if you feel 14 beats in six seconds your heart rate is 140 bpm.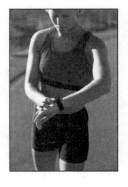

Remember, with PACE, **perceived exertion** is more important. There will be days when you don't achieve your usual heart rate. To use this example, if your maximum heart rate during exertion is 140 bpm, there will be times when you only hit 130 bpm. That's fine. It doesn't mean you're doing it wrong.

If you feel like you've pushed yourself and you've achieved heavy, fast and deep breathing, that is a successful PACE routine. That's perceived exertion – when you feel like you've given it everything you have. If your heart rate doesn't always match what you achieved during a previous session, that's fine.

> *"I've tried just about every diet and fitness program out there since I turned 16. And none of them were as easy as and worked as well as Dr. Sears'. When I started Dr. Sears' fat loss plan I weighed 169 lbs. and had 34% body fat. In the first month, I lost 7 lbs. and my body fat went down to 30%. Today I have lost a total of 19 lbs. so far and my body fat went down to 22%.*
>
> *I feel absolutely great! I went into my closet the other day and pulled out a bunch of dresses I used to wear years ago. And they all fit! I owe it all to Dr. Sears."*
>
> Eva J., Boynton Beach, FL

Recovery Time: Your *True* Measure of Heart Health

Recovery is one of the keys to successful PACE training. It's a lost art in our culture. Today, conventional exercise wisdom pushes you for long stretches of time without ever letting you catch your breath.

This is never the case in the natural world. As we've discussed, animals in the wild always exert themselves in short bursts followed by rest. So did ancient man.

This pattern of exertion followed by recovery is the basis of the body you have today. It's a pattern that's worked for hundreds of thousands, perhaps even millions of years. And the mechanism of benefit is clear. Recovery – or dynamic rest – is just that, it's *dynamic.*

When you rest and recover between exertion periods you're not wasting your time. Something vital and active is going on inside your body: *adaptive responses.*

Adaptive responses are the changes your body makes when it's given a challenge or a new stimulus. Your body makes adaptive responses all the time. The idea is to get your body to make the adaptive responses you want.

When you eat high-glycemic foods, your body makes an adaptive response by creating more insulin. Over time that will make you fat and put you at high risk for diabetes.

When you exercise aerobically, your body makes an adaptive response by shrinking your heart's output and lung capacity.

Both of these adaptive responses are clearly dangerous.

PACE is different. PACE encourages your body to make adaptive responses that are life-affirming. And it's during your recovery time that these changes start to take place. The German doctors and track coaches that invented interval training understood this. PACE takes it to the next level by making these responses available to you regardless of where you're starting. You don't need to be an Olympic athlete to get the benefits.

During your dynamic rest period you may not be "exercising," but your PACE program has set in motion a series of physiological changes that are quietly powering you to peak fitness:

- Your native afterburner kicks into gear, melting away the fat for hours after you finish your PACE routine.
- Your muscles refine their capacity for quick, powerful responses.

- Your pituitary gland triggers the release of youth-enhancing growth hormone.
- Your heart's output grows and becomes stronger, gradually adapting to develop greater reserve capacity and maximize the amount of blood it can pump with each beat.
- Your lung capacity expands to meet the new demand for more oxygen.

As you can see, what happens during recovery is just as important as what happens during exertion – if not more so. This is dynamic rest in action.

Track Your Recovery Time for a Stronger Heart and Robust Lungs

Keeping track of your recovery time is easy. After you finish your exertion period, stop and rest. Make note of the time. Take a drink of water and relax. Wait until you feel rested – until you feel like you've "caught your breath."

This is perceived recovery. In other words you rest until you feel like you've caught your breath. Make note of the time. How much time has elapsed? Three minutes? Ten minutes? There's no right or wrong answer here. Writing it down and keeping track is all you have to worry about.

Even if it takes you a long time to recover you can still make speedy progress with PACE. So don't be concerned.

A few years ago, I had a patient – JF – who was very out of shape. I put her on the treadmill at a low intensity. Within sixty seconds she was ready to fall over. I told her to stop and rest. After a full 5 minutes of recovery her heart was still beating at 140 bpm!

She was discouraged, but I told her not to worry about her results. I made sure she kept a log of her workouts and then followed up with her a few months later. *After 12 weeks, her heart was fully recovering from her exercise routine in just over two minutes.*

So keep a log and write everything down. After a few weeks when your body adapts and your heart strengthens, your recovery time will start to drop. (At the end of this book you'll find a website with log sheets you can download and print.)

Fast recovery is a sign of youth and vitality.

Children often have very fast recovery times. Because their hearts are young and resilient, they can run around at break-neck speed and be back to normal in seconds.

A few years ago, when my son was 5 or 6 years old, I had him run around the pool as fast as he could. I then measured his heart rate. It was an extremely fast 240 beats per minute. I measured again only 15 seconds later. It had returned to 120 bpm!

Watch for Warning Signs: Be Safe When You Practice PACE

Consult your doctor if your heart rate shows no sign of dropping within a few minutes of stopping exercise. Also see a doctor if you feel any of the following during exercise:

- An irregular or rapid heartbeat
- Light-headedness, dizziness or fainting
- Shortness of breath or chest pain

And please… always talk to your doctor before starting a new exercise routine.

How to Gauge Your Recovery Between Sets

Measuring your recovery time is easy enough. Simply make note of how long it takes your heart to return to normal after you exert yourself.

But what about between sets?

If you're doing four or five sets in your PACE routine, how far do you recover between sets? This is a common question.

When you finish your first set your recovery time will be faster than after you finish your fourth or fifth set. This is natural. After doing four sets your fatigue factor will be higher. And this will affect your recovery time.

> "I'm 92, and it is amazing to me and others that I am continually improving a little all of the time. I wonder if there are any records of an ol' guy like me continuing improvement over my age?"
>
> John M., Layton, UT

The fatigue that builds up after doing a number of sets is called *cumulative exertion*.

For example, after you finish one set you may feel winded but you probably won't feel fatigued. But after each successive set, you will feel increasingly worn out.

That means your recovery time between sets will vary. It will take you longer to recover after your fourth or fifth set than it will after your first set.

This is part of the process. Simply observe and take notes. Start your next exertion period after you feel like you've caught your breath. Rely on your sense of perceived recovery. When you've caught your breath and you feel rested you're ready to move on to the next set. Just don't wait around too long. You'll go cold.

The most important recovery time will be your last one. This is the amount of time it takes to recover from your last exertion period. This is the recovery time measurement that will give you your best gauge of progress.

The formula is very simple. As you become more conditioned your recovery time will come down. A shorter recovery time means your heart is stronger, healthier and more responsive.

Now that you have the tools to measure your progress, let's explore a deeper level of progressivity. This will give you an even deeper feeling of freedom and progress within your PACE program.

PATIENT STORY

Michael Masterson

"I dropped my skepticism when it started working for me..."

"I've seen Dr. Sears transform the lives of his patients for years. Many are friends of mine. But I was still a bit skeptical when he first told me about his 12-minute program.

That's why I'm so excited now. Not only have I experienced it for myself, I've seen other people do it too. And it just makes sense; the scientific proof behind it is logical and easy to understand.

The secret behind Dr. Sears' fat burning revolution is his PACE program. And when I put it to the test, I saw results almost immediately. Within a few weeks, I dropped 20 pounds of fat.

When I started PACE, I felt something new and quite remarkable: my lungs started to balloon inside my chest. I had never experienced anything quite like it before. I could begin to see the difference in my chest when I looked in the mirror. I felt like I could get twice the oxygen I was used to, I had more energy, and the benefits were long lasting.

Dr. Sears told me your lung capacity is your best indicator of 'all cause mortality.' That's doctor speak for 'all the ways you could possibly die.' In other words, the bigger your lung capacity, the longer you'll live. And I don't doubt it; extra oxygen has given me energy and an unshakable feeling of optimism.

Best of all, I didn't change my diet. Not a thing. I continue to enjoy all my favorites: steak, wine, cheese, seasonal fruits and vegetables, even the occasional dessert and cigar after dinner.

Life has never been better. And my friends are taking notice…
The fat around my belly is gone and my face looks young and lean."

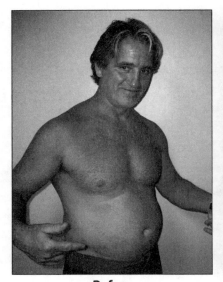
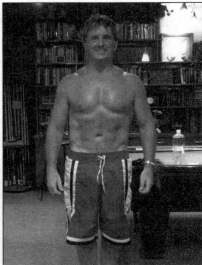

Before   **After**

CHAPTER EIGHT

Supercharge Your PACE

In a matter of weeks PACE will rebuild your native fitness. It will get and keep your heart pumping stronger, your lungs expanding and your muscles responding better for decades longer than current medical expectations.

Being effortlessly energetic with a naturally lean, high-performance body breeds stamina, power and confidence. It reconnects you to your environment and gives you back a keener sense of purpose.

Once you build native fitness you build and keep greater independence. You can call the shots and keep your mobility for life. Native fitness is the core of self-determination. Where others wind up bedridden or dependent, you're on the move. With the right plan, you take care of your body and it takes care of you.

When you challenge your body in the right way – in the way it was built to be challenged – it pays you back with greater vitality. It has been programmed to do so. With your vitality restored and sustained, you win back greater personal autonomy.

In case you're not old enough to fully appreciate the value of this possession, let me tell you from my experience in anti-aging therapies for the very elder – it's preciously rare yet priceless!

That's the gift that nature has programmed your body to give you… and it will… if you push the right buttons. Because these buttons were laid down and refined by millions of years of interaction with an environment now gone, this natural gift is lost. PACE will give it back.

Break Free of the Rigid Routines…
PACE Shatters All Convention

As you start your PACE program, you need to do something else different from what you are used to when you think of "exercise routines."

Aerobic classes and cardio workouts have two more things in common: they're both designed around fixed and repetitive movements. And they're both set on working your heart and lungs continuously for a set time period. That's the way we've been trained to move.

PACE breaks both these misguided traditions as well and puts you in touch with a principle that makes some people nervous at first. I'm talking about *change*. It's truly the only constant in the universe. It's the overriding rule of nature. And, our bodies thrive on it. But in the fitness world, it's often ignored or forgotten.

Repeating the same routine for an hour, mimicking the instructor in the same way every time, won't get you very far. Eventually it will start to injure you with useless wear and tear. You won't keep muscle and lose fat, and you won't save yourself from a heart attack.

PACE workouts are in a constant state of flux. They're not static. You never do it exactly the same way twice. And that scares some people. Most folks are creatures of habit and want to do things the same way every time. But that doesn't reflect the change inherent in nature. And it doesn't lead to native fitness.

PACE is not a form of aerobics or cardio. It's a different animal. And to practice PACE means listening to and accepting change.

When your body gets **used to** a particular challenge, it's **no longer challenging**. At that point you stop making

> *"I started PACE in late February and now am 25 lbs. lighter."*
> Clifford H., Pembroke Pines, FL

adaptive responses. You stop progressing. You will then be stuck "hitting a plateau." You're still spending the same time, doing the same work, but you're no longer moving forward. From a fitness improvement point of view, nothing is happening.

At this stage, you'll need to change gears and do something differently in your practice. By looking for this and listening to your body, you'll give yourself new challenges as the old ones become tired and predictable. In this way, PACE is never a chore; it's always new and exciting.

When you know the basic features of a PACE workout you can always change it up by altering the progressive element. By changing your workout, you're making creative solutions and breaking through plateaus.

This is different than what you might be used to. Traditional exercise doesn't always involve creativity. It doesn't ask you to contribute or listen. It simply demands the repetition of mechanical movements with no variation.

Let's review for a moment. We're talking about two key principles you'll be using as you continue your PACE practice:

- Recognizing the basic features of a PACE workout.
- Breaking through plateaus by applying a progressive element, i.e. – making incremental changes and applying creative solutions.

By now you're familiar with the basic features of a PACE workout: You give your body a worthy challenge, you hit your supra-aerobic zone during exertion, when you finish your exertion period you feel winded, you create an oxygen debt. You rest and recover. When you catch your breath you do another period of exertion.

These are the basic features you want to include in every PACE workout. How you do that is up to you. There are limitless possibilities. You can practice inside or outside. You can use an instrument or simply walk or run. You can do one set or you can do multiple sets.

This kind of freedom is both liberating and intimidating. If you can do anything, what do you choose?

In this chapter I'll provide you with some ideas. They will form the foundation of your PACE practice. But you'll add your own creative solutions as you progress. Recognizing when you've hit a plateau is part of the game.

Let's say you start off with one of the workouts you tried in Chapter 5. During the first couple of weeks you feel both challenged and rewarded. After each exertion period you feel winded and out of breath. You're monitoring and recording your maximum heart rate during exertion. You notice some improvement in your recovery time. You make small changes to your workout, like increasing the intensity, adding a set, etc.

These are all good signs.

But let's say after following this course for six weeks, the feeling starts to change. Your heart rate doesn't go as high... you don't feel as winded after each exertion period... you start to get bored... These are signs of reaching a plateau.

At that point you change your workout. You do something different. You apply the same basic features of PACE, but you do it in a new and creative way. That act of creative change brings back the exhilaration and it brings back the adaptive responses your body makes to a new challenge.

This is the key to a long-term successful PACE experience.

Below are some ideas with tips on what to do and what to look for...

PACE 8-Week Program

Weeks	Warm-Up	Set 1 Exertion	Set 1 Recovery	Set 2 Exertion	Set 2 Recovery
1 & 2	3 min	3 min	X min	3 min	X min
3 & 4	3 min	2 min	X min	2 min	X min
5 & 6	2 min	90 sec	X min	90 sec	X min
7 & 8	2 min	60 sec	X min	60 sec	X min

Weeks	Set 3 Exertion	Set 3 Recovery	Set 4 Exertion	Set 4 Recovery
1 & 2	3 min	X min	3 min	Done
3 & 4	2 min	X min	2 min	Done
5 & 6	90 sec	X min	90 sec	Done
7 & 8	60 sec	X min	60 sec	Done

> *"I have exercise-induced asthma. When I first started doing PACE, I needed to use my Albuterol inhaler afterwards each time. Within 3 weeks, I no longer needed to! I just took an introduction to a road cycling course. We rode 20 miles more than I've ever attempted before and while the few hills were hard, I didn't have any difficulty breathing."*
>
> Katie B., Benicia, CA

Here you have a basic 4-set workout. Every two weeks the exertion period decreases. To make it more challenging, you'll increase the intensity every time the exertion period gets smaller.

For example, let's say you choose an elliptical machine. Your first exertion period is three minutes so you set your incline at "4." The incline or the resistance settings will be different depending on what kind of machine you're using. But for the sake of example, let's say a setting of "4" is a low setting – something that will provide you a bit of a challenge but is not hard to maintain for three minutes.

The idea here is keeping your exertion level consistently high for three minutes, then resting. If your elliptical has a "strides per minute" read out, keep track of how high you get and what level gives you a feeling of exertion.

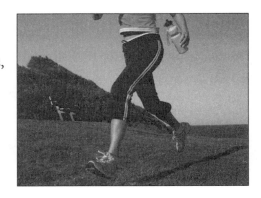

After two weeks, decrease the exertion period to two minutes. But make sure you increase the incline or intensity. Make it harder to do, but do it for a shorter period.

Play around with this workout but be mindful of the basic features of your PACE workout. Tailor it to suit your own level of conditioning.

Outdoor Running: Distance

Warm-Up	Set 1		Set 2	
	Exertion	Recovery	Exertion	Recovery
2 min	1/8 mile	X min	1/8 mile	X min

Set 3		Set 4	
Exertion	Recovery	Exertion	Recovery
100 yards	X min	100 yards	X min

Set 5		Set 6	
Exertion	Recovery	Exertion	Recovery
50 yards	X min	50 yards	Done

If you're in good condition, you can start your first exertion period by running an eighth of a mile (220 yards). Your intensity level should be moderate. After each recovery period, slightly increase the intensity. By the time you reach your 6th exertion period, you should be sprinting.

Here's a good variation: Run all six sets at 1/8 of a mile. The first three will feel easy. The last three will really test your stamina. If you can't sprint the entire way, that's fine. Do what you can and strive to give it a little extra effort each time you do it.

Here's yet another variation: Do this routine running uphill. This is a great workout. It's one of my personal favorites.

I'd like to draw your attention to an idea here… we're creating variations on a theme. This is an aspect of progressivity. As you practice a particular PACE workout consider different variations to keep it fresh.

Outdoor Running: Timed Exertion Periods

Warm-Up	Set 1		Set 2	
	Exertion	Recovery	Exertion	Recovery
1 min	2 min	X min	90 sec	X min

Set 3		Set 4	
Exertion	Recovery	Exertion	Recovery
60 sec	X min	45 sec	X min

Set 5		Set 6	
Exertion	Recovery	Exertion	Recovery
30 sec	X min	20 sec	Done

Like the distance program, start at a low to moderate intensity and increase the level of intensity after each set. The last two sets should be sprints.

When you're running outdoors, you can make it more difficult by running faster or running uphill. Your local area and terrain will determine which works best.

"It's a miracle. I weighed 121 lbs. my entire life until I turned 45. Then I started packing on the pounds – and I couldn't get the weight off! I had tried what seemed like thousands of diets. After I retired, I came to see Dr. Sears. I ended up losing 24 lbs., right off the bat! Now I'm remembering the good old days! I'm so happy; I could kiss Dr. Sears right now!"

Margaret V., Loxahatchee Groves, FL

Treadmill

Treadmills are a good option if walking or running outdoors isn't possible or convenient. You can raise intensity via speed or incline at the touch of a button. You also have the option of holding on to the side rails if you feel winded.

Begin walking at a comfortable pace for a few minutes until your muscles feel warm and loose. Increase the pace and lengthen your strides into a brisk walk, allowing your body to adapt. Start your first exertion period from this point. (Remember to wear proper running shoes with cushioned soles that absorb the impact of running.)

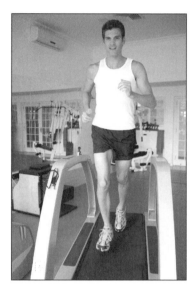

A sample treadmill PACE program will look similar to the outdoor, timed interval workout above – with a few slight variations. Bear in mind that it's easier to run fast or sprint when you're outside. When on a treadmill, I like to start and finish with a longer exertion period.

Having said that, experiment with this program and make it your own. If you apply the basic features of PACE, you have a lot of freedom. Use it.

Note: For treadmill programs, it is easy and works well to increase the intensity after each recovery period by slightly increasing your speed.

Here's another option: After you've steadily increased your

speed over a period of maybe four to six weeks, drop back to your original starting speed but increase the slope and repeat the entire cycle with the higher slope.

Warm-Up	Set 1		Set 2	
	Exertion	Recovery	Exertion	Recovery
1 min	3 min	X min	2 min	X min

Set 3		Set 4	
Exertion	Recovery	Exertion	Recovery
1 min	X min	1 min	X min

Set 5		Set 6	
Exertion	Recovery	Exertion	Recovery
2 min	X min	2 min	Done

Elliptical Machine

The elliptical trainer provides a high-energy, low-impact workout. This is a good option if you enjoy the feeling of running but don't like the pressure and impact on your knees.

Turning up the resistance on an elliptical triggers muscle growth in the quads and glutes (thighs and buttocks). At high levels it can be very demanding.

Most elliptical machines give you the option of adding an upper body workout. To work your arms, focus on pushing and pulling the handles; for more of a lower body workout, rest your hands on the handgrips, turn up the resistance and push harder with your legs.

After each recovery period, increase the incline so it takes more effort. You may want to hold on to the side rails for stability. Once you are used to this machine you can, for the last 2 exertion periods, run as fast as you can for 30 seconds each. You'll definitely feel the burn in your thighs.

One possible variation: Make each exertion period 2 minutes long. Your cumulative exertion will automatically make the last sets more difficult.

Note: To help you run faster, put the weight in the balls of your feet and lift your heels slightly. You can also raise your knees higher.

Warm-Up	Set 1		Set 2	
	Exertion	Recovery	Exertion	Recovery
2 min	2 min	X min	90 sec	X min

Set 3		Set 4	
Exertion	Recovery	Exertion	Recovery
60 sec	X min	40 sec	X min

Set 5		Set 6	
Exertion	Recovery	Exertion	Recovery
30 sec	X min	20 sec	Done

Stationary Bicycle or Recumbent Bicycle

When I'm in the gym, these two are my favorites. Both are great for working the larger muscles like the gluteus, quadriceps and the muscles of the lower back.

The stationary bike requires a little less effort, as your body is positioned over the pedals and your legs are pumping down. It also helps to improve your posture. Because both your hips and hands support your weight, your spine is in a horizontal position and gets a stretch in the lumbar region. The alternating hip motion created by your legs, works the muscles of the lower back, which affect your posture.

The recumbent bike is a good choice if you have edema (swelling) of the legs or problems with circulation. It also helps if you have lower back problems.

When exercising on a recumbent bike, you'll sit in a bucket seat and lean back against the backrest in a reclined position. The pedals on a recumbent bike are set horizontally in front of the seat, so your legs are straight out in front of you instead of below you. This puts less pressure on the joints, but makes resistance from the pedals a bit higher – giving you a more intense workout in a comfortable, natural position.

Warm-Up	Set 1		Set 2	
	Exertion	Recovery	Exertion	Recovery
2 min	2 min	X min	2 min	X min

Set 3		Set 4		Set 5	
Exertion	Recovery	Exertion	Recovery	Exertion	Recovery
90 sec	X min	60 sec	X min	60 sec	Done

This workout will challenge your endurance, so start at a low to moderate intensity. Increase the intensity as you progress. Feel the burn in your legs and take deep breaths making sure to exhale fully as the intervals shorten.

After a few weeks, turn up the heat and try the following program. The intervals are a bit shorter, so you should focus on intensity and maximum effort.

Warm-Up	Set 1		Set 2	
	Exertion	Recovery	Exertion	Recovery
2 min	1 min	X min	1 min	X min

Set 3		Set 4		Set 5	
Exertion	Recovery	Exertion	Recovery	Exertion	Recovery
30 sec	X min	20 sec	X min	20 sec	Done

Outdoor Bicycle

Like outdoor running, you can vary your routines with both distance and time. To vary intensity, look for paths and terrain that go both uphill and downhill. You can use flat, straight-aways to work with timed intervals, increasing your intensity by going faster. Depending on your bike, you can also change gears to make it harder or easier to pedal.

The workout is similar to outdoor running, except the exertion distances are longer to account for the speed of a bicycle. Biking is ideal if you're overweight; it's an exceptional fat burner and there's no impact to injure joints.

"My story is only beginning, but I'm so excited, I had to write. I was at my ideal weight 2 1/2 years ago, but then went through menopause and gained 26 lbs. despite constant attempts at modifying my diet and exercise routine.

I only started PACE five days ago, have had three workouts on a stationary bicycle, and have already lost 3 lbs., 2 1/2 inches around my waist, 1 inch off my hips, 1 inch off my bust, and 1 inch off of each thigh. And my resting heartbeat has dropped by a full 10 beats!!"

Gia B., Los Angeles, CA

Outdoor Bicycle: Brief Measured Distance Program

Warm-Up	Set 1		Set 2	
	Exertion	Recovery	Exertion	Recovery
2 min	1 mile	X min	1 mile	X min

Set 3		Set 4	
Exertion	Recovery	Exertion	Recovery
1/2 mile	X min	1/2 mile	X min

Set 5		Set 6	
Exertion	Recovery	Exertion	Recovery
1/4 mile	X min	1/8 mile	Done

Outdoor Bicycle: Longer Timed Exertion Periods

Warm-Up	Set 1		Set 2	
	Exertion	Recovery	Exertion	Recovery
2 min	4 min	X min	4 min	X min

Set 3		Set 4	
Exertion	Recovery	Exertion	Recovery
3 min	X min	3 min	X min

Set 5		Set 6	
Exertion	Recovery	Exertion	Recovery
2 min	X min	1 min	Done

As with all of these workouts, *experiment.* By now you understand that PACE is the dynamic or creative application of a few basic principles. As long as you achieve the basics during each routine, the exertion periods can be as long or as short as you like.

Just bear one thing in mind…

Keep Your Total Exertion Under 20 Minutes

I often refer to PACE as the "12-minute fitness revolution." In my experience I've found 12 minutes of total exertion is enough to trigger the adaptive responses we've talked about.

By "12 minutes of total exertion" I mean that all your exertion periods add up to 12 minutes. So if you do four sets of three minutes each, that's 12 minutes of total exertion.

While 12 minutes is a good PACE workout, you can certainly go beyond that if you like. Just keep your total exertion time under 20 minutes. You can do as many sets as you like, but the total amount of exertion for the workout should not go over 20 minutes.

For example, if you did six sets of four minutes each, that would equal 24 minutes of total exertion. That's a bit too long for a PACE workout. Why? It's about fuel. As you've learned, your body changes its fuel sources. During the first few minutes, you're burning ATP supplied by your cells. Then you switch gears and burn carbs from your muscle tissue. Finally, after about 20 minutes you start burning fat.

Remember… you don't want to burn fat *during* your workout. That's why you never exceed 20 minutes of total exertion. After your PACE workout is *finished*, your body will replenish your muscle tissue by burning your fat stores. This fat burning goes on for hours after you finish, even while you're sleeping.

PATIENT STORY

Carlos Menendez

Coach Scott, my PACE-certified fitness trainer, brought Carlos to our clinic after meeting him at the gym. Scott felt like Carlos was a great candidate for PACE.

When the two met, Carlos was trying to get back in shape after "letting it slide" for a number of years. Like many guys, Carlos was very active in his 20s but fell out of his fitness routine when the demands of his career and family got to be too much.

Being a talented soccer player, Carlos was eager to get back in the game. And he responded to PACE quickly and with a lot of enthusiasm.

In his "after" picture, Carlos looks about 10 years younger.

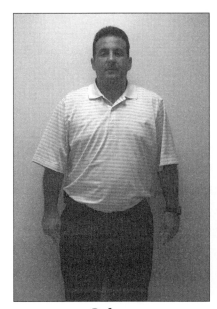 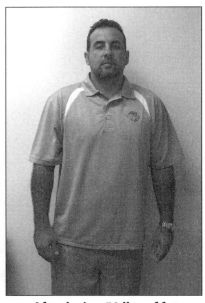

Before   **After losing 50 lbs. of fat**

As of this writing, Carlos has been doing PACE for six months. In that time, he:

- Lost 50 pounds of fat
- Built 29 pounds of new muscle
- Raised HDL (good cholesterol) by over 65%
- Lowered triglycerides (blood fat) by over 10%

Body Fat (lbs)

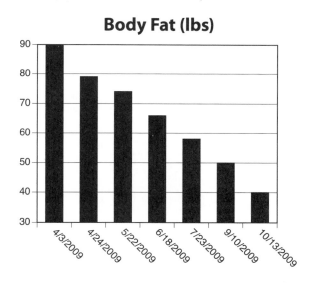

Lean Body Mass (lbs)

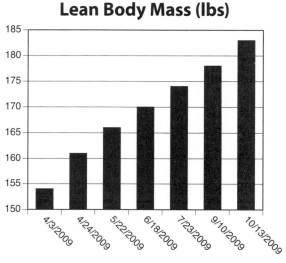

HDL (mg/dL)

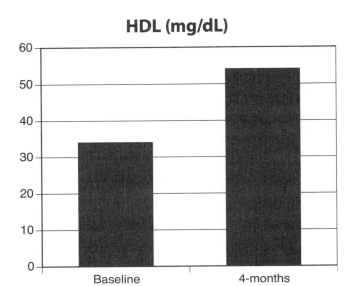

Triglycerides (mg/dL)

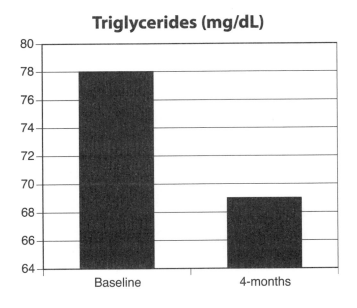

www.pacerevolution.com

CHAPTER NINE

Rebuild Real Strength

Now that you are well on your way to building real strength and power in your heart and lungs, it's time to ask a related question: What about muscle strength?

Your muscles have a problem very much like the problem I exposed with heart and lung strength. These problems are similar in two ways. First, our environment is no longer providing the challenges to our muscles that we were designed to get from our daily activities. Second, you can't count on conventional advice to solve this problem.

If you go to the average gym today and tell the staff that you want to get stronger, they're probably going to tell you to lift weights – right? But if you want real strength that you can use, forget lifting weights. And those machines with cables or rubber bands are even worse.

Weight lifting is the best exercise for creating muscle bulk, but isn't so good for building real strength that you can use. Weight lifters look impressive because they have created *muscle hypertrophy*. But big muscles are a cosmetic feature.

Indeed when we look at practical strength tests we find that strength and hypertrophy are very much different and are produced with different training programs. In fact, if you watch very hypertrophied bodybuilders play sports they're unusually tight, clumsy and awkward. The muscle development they work so hard for actually gets in their way.

"PACE Strength" Keeps You Nimble, Fast and Youthful

Muscle hypertrophy, or the increase in muscle cell size, is the prize of most body builders. But there are actually two forms of hypertrophy: one that leads to size but not strength, and one that translates into real muscular strength you can use.

Sarcoplasmic hypertrophy is the rise of sarcoplasmic fluid in the muscle cell but with no increase in muscular strength. This is typical of most body builders. *Myofibrillar hypertrophy* is the increase of contractile proteins, which builds muscular strength but with a smaller increase in the muscle size. This is typical of most strength trainers.[1]

> "I loved the PACE book and am into my second week. Congratulations. There's hope for the elderly."
>
> Tom R., Antigonish, Nova Scotia, Canada

PACE encourages myofibrillar hypertrophy, the kind that builds real strength. To get there, you focus on ***progressively increasing*** your challenge to continuously stress the contractile proteins.[2]

While body builders may appear to have more size, sarcoplasmic hypertrophy is achieved by exhausting the muscles to the point where they are fatigued and unable to move.[3] Not what you want for long-term health, strength and mobility.

Functional strength on the other hand, is practical strength. It keeps you nimble, fast and youthful. It's what enables you to climb the stairs while you're carrying four bags of groceries without injuring yourself.

Functional strength propels you out of bed in the morning and helps you carry out life's daily tasks. And as you get older, functional strength keeps you mobile, independent, and out of the nursing home until the day you arrive at the Pearly Gates.

As you are doing PACE you're working on functional strength training. It's one of the benefits activated every time you do PACE. You can further improve your functional strength training with PACE by making a few simple variations. You can use your own body weight to focus your training on specific muscle groups.

In this way you'll not only make progress faster but you will ultimately reach a level of power, strength and competency you never imagined possible. And you can keep this level of confidence and fitness as you age.

In this chapter I'll show you how. It's not as hard as you might think. And it never feels like a chore. By the time you finish your first challenge you'll feel exhilarated and recharged.

Weight Training Doesn't *Train* Anything... Except the Risk of Injury

Rarely is muscle hypertrophy alone the goal of my training programs. In those uncommon cases progressive weight training to near exhaustion is the best tool for the job. If done properly, it will cause your muscle to enlarge. But even then it is best combined with some type of more functional strength training.

In all my years as a personal trainer, coach, fitness consultant and anti-aging physician I can't escape one more very negative limitation of weight training – you're not really *training* anything. What you're actually doing is conditioning your muscles to tense up, tearing fibers and creating bloated hypertrophied muscle fibers in response.

This new muscle mass becomes dysfunctional because it's disconnected from the central nervous system's primary purpose of muscle control – to work with other muscles to move your body.

Long-term weight lifting creates strength, tension and size imbalances, unnatural patterns of movement, malpositioned joints and sets you up for injuries. And it's certainly not the best way to build *functional* strength you can use.

What's more, your body isn't designed for the mechanics of weight lifting patterns. For someone with low muscle mass, a well-designed lower body resistance workout can help restore the lost muscle mass. But for many in my clinic, the recurrent unnatural strain has produced too many injuries.

Aside from the widespread and well-known weight lifting injuries like torn muscles and trauma to the rotator cuff, elbows, knees and lower back, weight lifting has a darker, more dangerous side to it. And much of it is still emerging.

In 2003, surgeons at Yale-New Haven Hospital first discovered a potentially fatal danger for weight lifters. Blood pressure, which is usually 120/80, rose to levels of 300

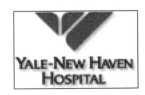

www.pacerevolution.com

or higher for people who bench pressed weights equal to their own body weight.[4]

Keep in mind, for the average weight lifter, bench-pressing their own body weight is considered to be a moderate challenge at best. An accomplished body builder can routinely bench-press twice their body weight or more.

After seeing five young patients with heart damage following weight lifting, the Yale researchers concluded the intense pressure led to ruptures of the internal layer of the aorta, called *aortic dissection*. This tearing of the lining of the largest blood vessel in the body is fatal unless treated immediately. Their study, published in *JAMA*, the *Journal of the American Medical Association,* was followed up three years later with more evidence and a direct warning.

This time the Yale surgeons called for widespread heart screenings of anyone considering weight lifting.[5] Their follow up results, published in the journal *Cardiology*, were summed up by lead surgeon and researcher Dr. John Elefteriades:

"Of the 31 patients, 10 of them are dead." [6]

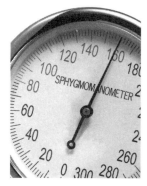

Their discovery is tragic but not surprising. Repetitive heavy lifting to the point of exhaustion isn't natural to our bodies. We weren't designed for that kind of exertion. Pumping your muscles for the sake of size and not strength can lead to trouble.

Nature designed your body to build and maintain muscle in response to the demands of your own body weight. "Exercising" this natural function, i.e. – moving your body weight – is also the most effective way to strengthen ligaments and tendons.

Turn on the Top 8 Benefits of Strong Muscles

Once you combine PACE with a strength-training program, these eight health enhancers turn on like a switch:

1. Lower resting blood pressure.

2. Reduction of body fat.

3. Reduction of symptoms associated with Type II diabetes: depression, sleep disorders, osteoporosis and depression.

4. Muscle strength is increased and muscle loss is prevented.

5. Increased bone mass and density to protect against osteoporosis, a disease that affects bone fragility.

6. Alleviates lower back pain and increases lower back strength.

7. Improves functional flexibility and strength, keeping you safe during daily activities.

8. Improves personal appearance, physique, self-esteem and self-confidence.

Reference: Ross J. Strength Training for Seniors.
The American College of Sports Medicine. 2004

Power Up New Muscle Strength With Nature's Fitness Trainer

Before the modern fads of aerobics, cardio and weight lifting took over and created the commercialized modern gym, going to the gym used to mean boxing, wrestling, push-ups, chin-ups and calisthenics.

After trying it all myself and testing and researching strength building for 30 years, the best way to build the kind of functional strength that you use in normal daily activities remains exercises that use your own body weight. Bodyweight exercises are a type of "functional exercise" because they train function or real world use. They employ positions and motions that you use to move your own body. In this way they mimic the challenges that we were designed to face but now lack in the modern world.

This recent trend in muscle strengthening science – away from weight training and toward body weight exercise – is really not new at all but simply returning to an earlier more natural and wiser method. In fact, you could call most functional, bodyweight exercises good old-fashioned *calisthenics*.

The Greek word "calisthenics" comes from "kallos" for beauty and "thenos" for strength. Practiced over time, they make it easier to perform routine physical tasks, and they improve bone density, metabolism and immune function. They have long been at the core of the strength-training program for the U.S. Green Berets and Navy Seals.

> *"I am now completing my 'rookie year' as a cop and at 60, I am fully able to handle the daily rigors of the job. I owe most of that to PACE."*
>
> Mark P., Liberty, MO

The good news is that you are already addressing muscle strength with PACE. Because all my PACE programs employ your body weight in natural movements, you will be building real muscle strength. With a little variation you can use different calisthenics to challenge different muscle groups in functional patterns to generate considerable muscle strength.

You can do calisthenics whether you're on the road, in the office, or at home. It's the perfect "anytime, anywhere" exercise. No special or expensive equipment is necessary and with a few simple maneuvers, you can exercise multiple muscle groups.

As with any exercise program, begin slowly. In just a few weeks, you should see results if you remain consistent and stay with the program. You'll need to build up your stamina by starting slowly and increasing your endurance.

Speed Your Recovery From Heart Attack and Heart Disease

People of all ages benefit from muscular conditioning, especially those needing to recover from heart disease.

As we get older, muscle wasting causes us to lose the ability to move our bodies, often requiring the assistance of walking aids and wheelchairs. By increasing the size of your muscles, you also improve your stamina and stability.

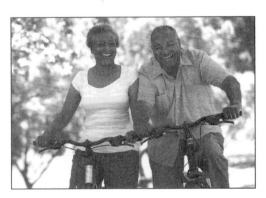

Using a functional resistance-training program, such as calisthenics, is your best approach to muscle conditioning. Strengthening your muscle capacity creates *positive muscle adaptation*. This makes performing everyday physical activities *less* challenging.

I like to begin with several repetitions of arm circles, leg lifts, upper body rotations, and hurdle steps. Moving your body through these physical motions will prevent injury by loosening joints and tendons.

Here's How You Do It: More Power and More Strength in 3 Easy Steps

PACE gets results by adding a progressive element to your

workout. It doesn't matter if you're walking, riding a bike or running on a treadmill. Calisthenics are no different.

My favorite strategy is simple: Time yourself and try and do it faster next time.

Start by selecting three calisthenics or body-weight exercises. I like to start with:

- Jump Squats
- Jump Pull-Ups
- Push-Ups

When you're ready, do 100 repetitions of each. Time yourself. If you need to take a break that's fine. As soon as you are able to get going again, pick up the count where you left off.

Here's an example: You look at your watch or use a stopwatch. You start with jump squats. You do 30 without a break. You stop and rest. You do another 40 and then rest again. You do 30 more then rest. Then you start your jump pull-ups. You keep going in spurts until you finish. You do the same with push-ups. Now... you're done.

How long did it take you? Twenty minutes? Forty minutes? An hour? It doesn't matter. As long you time yourself and do 100 of each.

Now here's the progressive element of this training program. Next time, you time yourself again and shoot for doing it *a little faster each time.*

This is a simple yet very effective way of doing PACE with calisthenics. You're working all the major muscle groups in a way that promotes strength, coordination and new myofibril growth. And by challenging yourself to do it slightly faster each time, you're using the PACE techniques of progressivity and acceleration.

You are more likely to make progressive changes if you keep a detailed report, make note of how long it takes to do each exercise. The first time I did this routine it took me about 15 minutes: Four minutes for the jump squats, 4 minutes for the jump pull-ups and 3 minutes for the push-ups... and about 4 minutes of rest in between.

It's helpful if you record your heart rate at each stage too. You'll be able to monitor your progress more effectively.

Remember: take it slow. It doesn't matter how long it takes; especially at the beginning. Be patient and be diligent.

> *"I love PACE. I have had a lot of success with the program. My clothes are big on me!!! Yippee!"*
> Sharon B., Boynton Beach, FL

For descriptions of the exercises, see below. (If you get too tired doing normal push-ups, try doing wall push-ups or knee push-ups.)

Looking for variations or new ideas? The three exercises mentioned above work brilliantly together. But you can use others. Try choosing one routine from each category below to make a new challenge.

Here's an example:

- Alternating Lunges, 100 repetitions
- Crunches, 100 repetitions
- Dips, 100 repetitions

There are infinite possibilities here. For new challenges, combine with other calisthenics mentioned in this chapter.

Stay Independent and Mobile as You Age

✓ **No Wheelchairs**
✓ **No Dependence on Others**
✓ **No Assisted Living Facilities**

Don't give up control over your own life. PACE keeps you functional in these key areas:

MOVE	CARRY	PICK UP	GET UP	ENDURE
Climb stairs	Groceries	Packages	Out of the car	In the hot sun
Walk about	Luggage	Children	Out of bed	In the cold wind
Run for cover	Supplies	Boxes	Off the couch	On long travels
				On endless shopping trips

Lower Body Strength: Your Key to Life-Long Mobility

Here's another point you are unlikely to hear from your gym: when it comes to restoring your native strength, your lower body needs more attention than your upper body. These muscles are bigger and meant to be stronger. In our native world they would bear the biggest challenges but are the most neglected in our modern world. They provide your foundation and you should focus on strengthening them first.

Your three biggest muscles work to flex and extend your hip joint. These muscles are:

- Quadriceps on the front of your thighs.
- Hamstrings on the back of your thighs.
- Gluteus muscles in your buttocks.

Four of the best exercises for these muscles are:

- **Hindu Squats** – Stand with your feet shoulder-width apart. Extend your arms out in front of you, parallel to the ground with your hands open and palms facing down. Inhale briskly and pull your hands straight back. As you pull back, turn the wrists up and make a fist. At the end of the inhalation, your elbows should be behind you with both hands in a fist, palm side up.

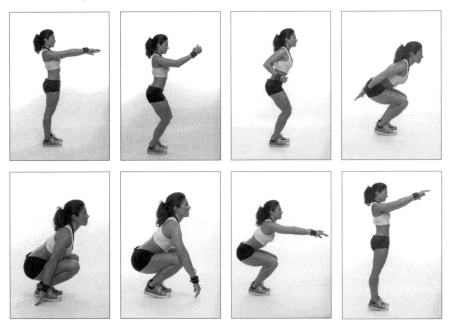

From this position, exhale, bend your knees and squat. Let your arms fall to your sides and touch the ground with the tips of your fingers. Continue exhaling and let your arms swing up as you stand.

This brings you back to the starting position: standing straight up with your arms extended in front of you, hands open and palms facing down.

Repeat at the pace of one repetition every four seconds. Once you are comfortable with the form, you can increase your speed to one squat per second.

Repeat until you feel winded. Rest, recover and do another set. Once you're conditioned, you'll be able to do 100 repetitions in a set. (I do 500 every other day...)

- **Alternating Lunges** – With your hands on your hips, take a step forward with your right leg until your front knee is bent 90 degrees and your back knee almost touches the ground. Push off from your leading foot and return to the starting position. Repeat with your left leg.

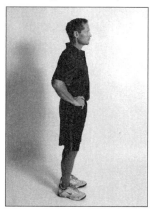 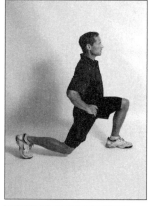

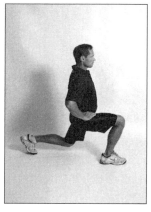 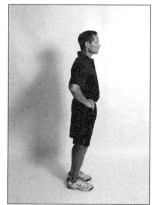

- **Squats** – With feet shoulder width apart, squat as far as possible. Bring your arms forward, parallel to the floor. Return to standing position. Repeat.

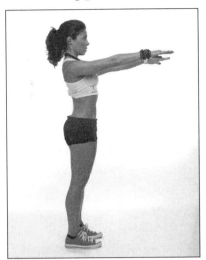 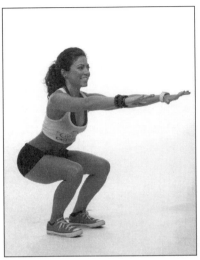

- **Jump Squats** – With body crouched, feet together, arms at sides, head straight and level, quickly straighten legs and jump upward as high as you can. Simultaneously, extend arms and reach overhead. After landing, quickly return to original position, without losing your balance. Repeat.

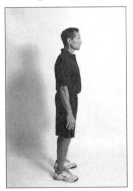 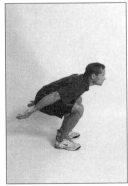 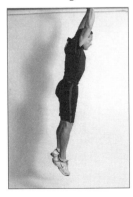

Begin with these muscles and work them first if you want to maximize the effect on your total body strength.

Easily Maintain Rock-Hard Abs
and Wipe Out Lower Back Pain

To prevent pain and injury in the lower back, you must have strong abdominal muscles. Functional strength is supported by building powerful core muscle groups to improve your breath, posture, and mechanics of motion. The four best floor exercises for concentrating on your abdomen include:

- **Crunches/Sit-Ups** – Lie on your back, raise your head and feet slightly, hold, and repeat.

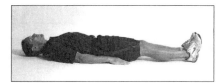 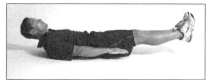

- **Leg Levers** – Lie on your back, legs six inches off the ground. Lift legs another foot higher, return to starting position. Repeat.

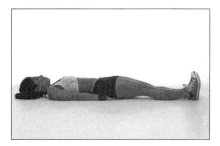 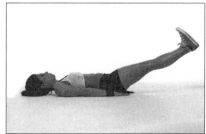

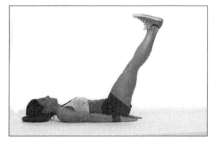 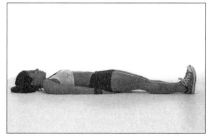

- **Back Flutter Kicks** – Lie on your back, and alternate each leg 2 to 3 feet off ground. Repeat.

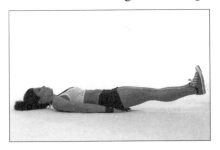
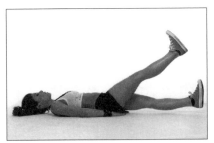

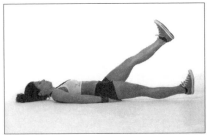
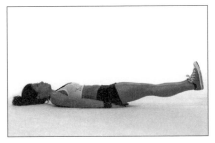

- **Scissors** – Lie on your back, raise legs a few inches off ground. Spread legs apart and then bring them together. Repeat.

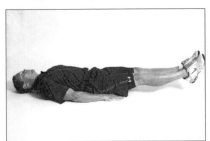
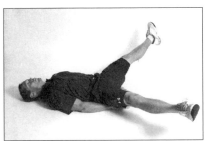

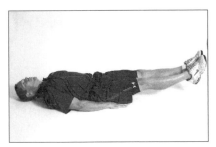
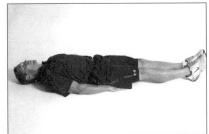

Pump Up Your Chest and Arms
Without Going to the Gym

You build practical strength by engaging in a full range of motion activities. Challenge your upper body by using your own body weight. Everyday activities, like lifting heavy packages or moving furniture, will be easier as your muscles build useful strength.

To prevent injury, focus more on your back than your chest and arms. The best exercises for building upper body strength include:

- **Push-Ups** – Lie face down. Place hands a little wider than shoulder-width apart. Straighten your back and place feet together. Lower yourself until you almost touch the ground.

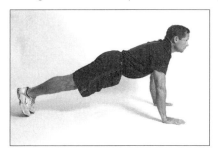 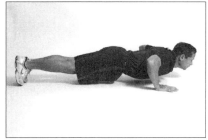

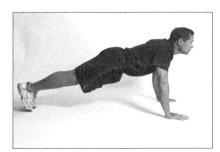 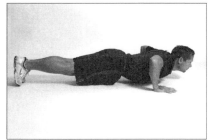

- **Wall Push-Up (Modified Push-Up)** – This exercise is great for people who are not able to do a regular push up. Start standing up and then lean against a wall with your hands out. Now with your hands at shoulder length apart lower yourself toward the wall. Now press your body back to the starting position. To make it more challenging find something lower like a desk or bench.

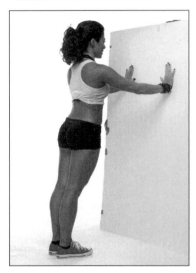 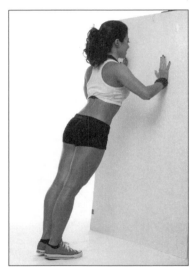

- **Knee Push-Up (Modified Push-Up)** – Start with your knees on the floor and your feet up. Place your hands parallel with your shoulders and a bit wider than shoulder-width apart. Extend your arms until your arms come close to locking out. Lower yourself until you almost touch the ground. Repeat.

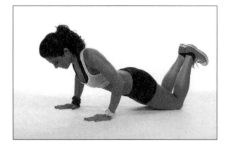 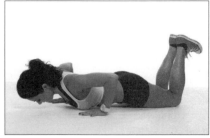

- **Arm Haulers** – Lie on your stomach. Stretch your arms in front of you. Raise arms and legs off floor and sweep arms back to your thighs (similar to a breaststroke). Return arms to starting position. Repeat.

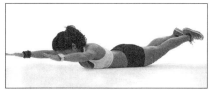 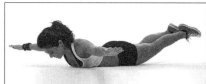

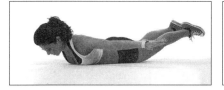 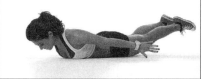

- **Pull-Ups** – Palms face out for a traditional pull-up on a bar to strengthen middle back muscles. Palms face toward you to do a chin-up, which strengthens the back and biceps.

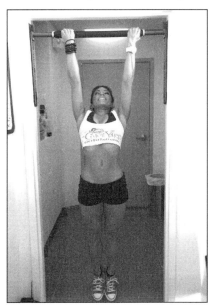 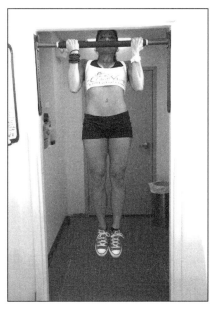

- **Jump Pull-Ups** – Same as above except you start with your feet on the floor. Your hands are on the bar as you would for a normal pull-up, but with your knees slightly bent. Jump up with your legs and pull yourself up at the same time. Jumping with your legs gives you more power and lets you do more repetitions than if your body were hanging from the bar.

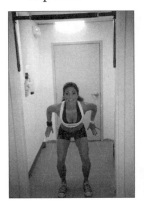 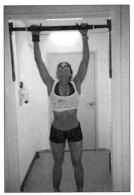 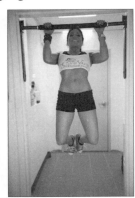

- **Dips** – Use parallel bars, two chairs or two desks. Lift feet off ground, while putting one hand on each object. Slowly lower yourself until elbows are at 90-degree angles. Pause. Slowly raise yourself. Repeat. Excellent exercise for chest, middle back and triceps.

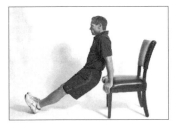 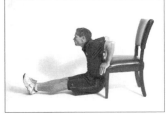
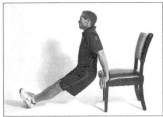 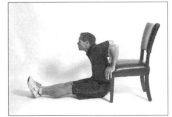

You can alternate with these other bodyweight exercises:

- **Instep Touches** – Stand with feet shoulder-width apart, toes slightly pointing outward, arms extended to your sides and parallel to the floor, head straight and level. Bend forward at your waist, turn your upper body, and bring the fingers of one hand to instep of opposite foot. Keep arms and legs straight but not locked. Simultaneously, raise your other arm to ceiling. Repeat.

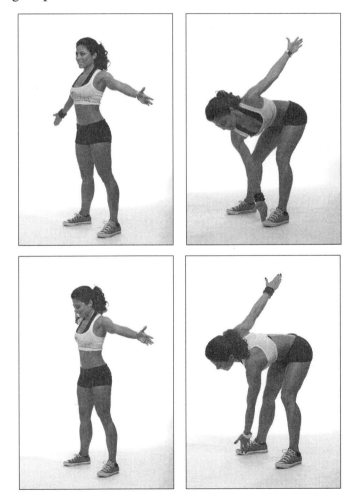

- **Knee Bends** – With feet almost together and arms at sides, head straight and level, bend your knees to lower your body. When thighs are parallel, rise up on your toes, while simultaneously swinging your arms forward. Your arms will be parallel to the floor in front of you, with fingers together and palms facing down and back, remaining perpendicular to the floor. Reverse this motion, without stopping, and return to original starting position. Repeat.

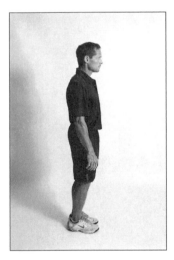 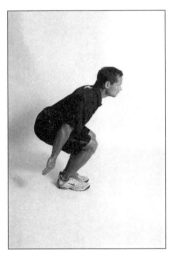

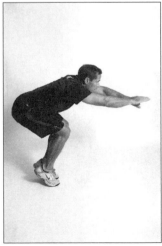 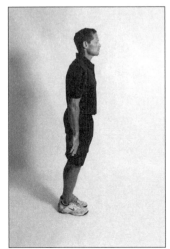

Or you can try a few of these ***plyometric*** exercises. Plyometrics training is designed to produce fast, powerful movements. Used for athletic and sports performance, plyometric exercise enhances the nervous system and allows for higher jumps, faster sprints and farther throws.

Applied to PACE and functional strength, plyometric exercises build strength, power and range of movement – especially in the lower body, which provides you with the "getting up" and "climbing" ability.

- **Jump to Box** – In this exercise a "box" can be a platform, a bench or a piece of gym equipment that provides a "step up" of several inches up to a couple of feet. Stand facing the box with your feet a bit wider than shoulder-width. Lower your body into a half-squat position and immediately jump up onto box. Don't pause or wait too long in your squat position before jumping. Your feet should land softly on box. After you jump, step back down to the ground; don't jump back down. Repeat.

- **Tuck Jumps** – This movement is basically a jump into the air as high as you can while bringing your legs in and your knees up to your chest. Stand with your feet shoulder-width apart; keep your knees slightly bent and your arms at your sides. Jump up bringing your knees up to your chest. Land on balls of feet and repeat immediately. Stay on the ground for as little time as possible before repeating. Remember to land soft on feet and spring back into the air.

- **Bounding** – This movement resembles a big leap while running. Think of a long-distance jumper right before he launches himself… like a gazelle darting through the bush. Start

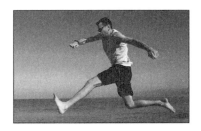

by jogging to gain forward momentum. When you're ready, forcefully push off with the left foot. At the same time, move your right arm forward. Repeat with the other leg and arm. Think of an exaggerated running motion and focus on your push-off and air time.

- **Bounding with Rings** – Same as above except that you put rings on the ground. As you push off your foot, you land in the rings, which are 3 to 4 feet out on either side.

- **Box Drill with Rings** – This movement involves jumping from side to side with 4 rings placed in the form of a square. Start by standing with your feet slightly wider than hip-width apart in the first circle. Hop forward using both feet and land in second ring right in front of you. Now hop to the left and land in the ring to your left side. Now jump backward to land in ring behind you. Finish by jumping to your right to land in the ring you started in. Rest and repeat.

Note: For demonstrations of the plyometric routines, refer to your PACE video. (See Appendix A.)

If you feel any dizziness, shortness of breath or pain, slow down. Do not over-exert yourself. If done effectively, you will transform your body through the power of calisthenics. By doing a regular calisthenics routine, you'll see improvements in your stamina and appearance.

Endnotes

1 Zatsiorsky VM, Kraemer WJ. Science and Practice of Strength Training. *Human Kinetics*. 2006. Champaign, IL.

2 Ibid

3 Ibid

4 Elefteriades JA, Hatzaras I, Tranquilli MA, et al. Weight Lifting and Rupture of Silent Aortic Aneurysms. *JAMA*. 2003;290(21):2803

5 Hatzaras I, Tranquilli M, Coady PM, et al. Weight Lifting and Aortic Dissection: More Evidence for a Connection. *Cardiology*. 2007;107:103-106

6 Gramza J. Weightlifting Death Risk. *ScienCentral*. Jul 18, 2006.

Rik Pavlescak

Rik came to my office in December of 2006 and told me he felt okay in general but had trouble losing weight and keeping it off.

During that first consultation we did a round of blood testing and talked about a plan of action. He showed an immediate interest in PACE and felt like it could work. After the holiday break he returned in January of 2007 to start PACE.

Rik's progress was swift and dramatic. In just three months, Rik:

- Lost 48 pounds of fat
- Built 24 pounds of new muscle
- Lowered his triglycerides (blood fat) from 470 to 256

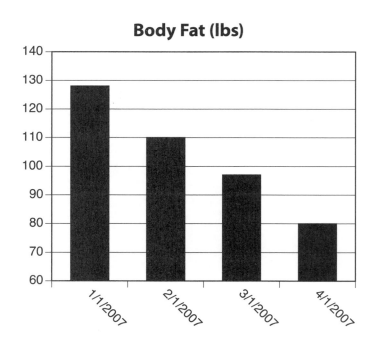

Body Fat (lbs)

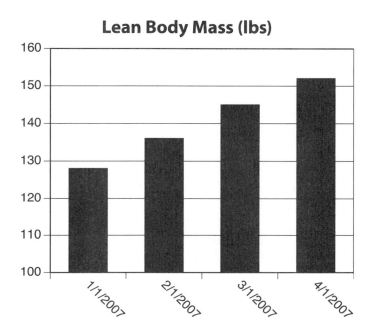

Lean Body Mass (lbs)

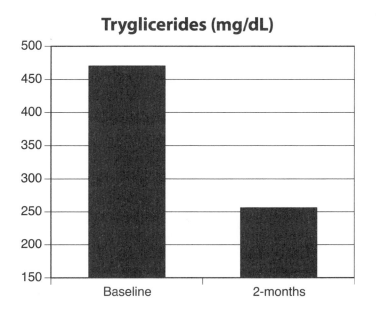

Tryglicerides (mg/dL)

Rik is another example of PACE delivering fast results.

His pictures tell the whole story.

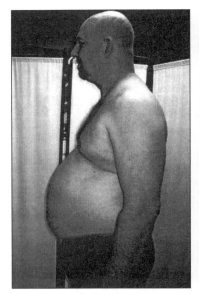 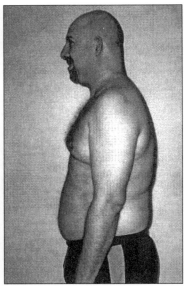

Rik Before   **Rik with 48 lbs. less fat**

CHAPTER TEN

Stay Lean for Life

Power Your PACE With Foods You Love

PACE naturally burns fat, builds muscle, expands your lungs and bulletproofs your heart. But each one of these natural capacities comes faster and easier when you start eating the foods you were born to eat.

Once again, just like with our routine physical challenges, the modern world changed our eating habits as well. It happened without our full knowledge or consent. We are simply born into it. And once again the modern medical establishment and popular media failed to recognize the real problem and prescribed the wrong solutions.

In fact, all the bird food, tofu burgers and low-fat garbage that tastes likes cardboard are no better than the other unnatural processed junk food they are designed to replace. It's all substitute food when what we really need is simply the same stuff we always ate for many millennia – I'm talking about real food: salty red meats, fresh eggs, fish, raw vegetables and sweet fruits.

In this chapter I'll put these myths to rest. I'll show you how to quickly hit and maintain your ideal weight. And, you won't have to suffer through one more day of bland, tasteless food.

As you'll discover, your ancestors didn't fret about fat or count calories. They enjoyed naturally lean and muscular bodies by following their instincts. You can too. It's easier than you think.

Fat Loss Myth #1: Counting Calories Is the Best Way to Burn Fat

Doctors and nutritionists would have you believe that counting calories is the only way to lose fat. How many times have you heard this misguided advice?

- Calories in, calories out… that's all you need to worry about.
- If you consume more calories than you burn, the rest turns to fat.
- The best way to burn calories is aerobic exercise.

There's only one problem. Their theory seems to make sense but it almost always fails when you try to apply it in the real world. It just doesn't work. Your body is not a machine. It's a living, sentient being that has its own "intelligence." It reacts to what it judges its environment to be. It decides on its own how to use the calories you consume. I propose that excess calories do not automatically turn to fat.

Of course, some people just eat way too much. If you're trying to lose fat, such over consumption will obviously get in your way. But for most people trying to lose weight that's not the problem. And for the majority of people, I tell them: If you want to lose fat and keep it off, forget about calories.

You may be surprised to hear that. It may sound like a contradiction. Let me explain why I believe counting calories is not necessary or even very helpful in losing fat. I will show you in the same way I learned – from a patient's story.

This point is one I was regrettably slow to learn. I thought it violated the laws of thermodynamics, so I had to be beaten over the head with it before it finally sank in.

Eating Fewer Calories and Getting Heavier By the Day

A young woman came to my clinic about 17 years ago. We'll call her LS. She was 5′ 2″ and weighed 170 pounds. She had been trying to lose weight for two years but said, *"No matter how little I eat, my weight just keeps going up."*

When I asked her about exercise, she insisted, *"I work as a waitress and I'm on the run for 10 hours a day. And I'm up to working out 5 times a week."*

I told her to cut her calories to 1600 and see me in 2 weeks. She did this diligently and brought me a complete record. Her weight went up by 4 pounds. I told her to bring down her calories to 1400 per day. The result? She gained four more pounds.

I cut her to 1200 then 1000 calories and again she gained weight. Now she lacked energy,

"I've tried 11 years of weight loss diets and nothing seemed to work. I'd take off the weight and once I stopped the diet, my weight would creep up again. I went to see Dr. Sears and his weight loss program was so easy, I adapted quickly. I was wearing an extra, extra large and now I wear a medium. I weighed 210 lbs. and I now weigh 170 lbs. Everyone has noticed my weight loss and I'm so full of energy that I'm doing things now that I couldn't do before."

Barbara S., Boca Raton, FL

couldn't make herself go to the gym anymore, and was feeling depressed.

She still wanted to lose weight. So… I told her to cut her calories to 800 and see me again in 2 weeks. I never saw her again and she didn't return the calls from my office. If I could, I would apologize to her and tell her what we did wrong.

Sticking to the Wrong Strategy for Weight Loss

You have probably heard that conventional diets don't work. History has shown that 5 out of 6 people who try to lose weight fail. And more than 90% of those who do succeed in losing weight gain all the weight back within 2 years.

When you consider the flawed strategy these diets use, this is no surprise. It's exceptionally difficult to stay healthy and achieve and maintain your ideal weight by starving yourself thin. Even if you could do it, it would eventually rob you of the very things that make life sweet.

Losing weight has been so hard because you have the wrong tool for the job. If you drop your calories too low and go hungry – forcing your body to lose weight – your body will fight you in this effort. Remember, your body has a built in "intelligence."

It reacts as if you are starving and will do everything it can to preserve your fat. And when you lose weight through starving yourself, you also lose important muscle, bone and even vital organ mass.

Your body has mechanisms for setting your weight at where it wants it to be. It is similar to the way you set your house temperature with your thermostat.

So the right tool for the job is one that changes your set point. The good news is that you can change the controls for your set point. But they're not the diet and exercise that we used to think. They involve eating differently – not necessarily eating less.

Pushing 5,000 Calories a Day and Still Dropping Pounds

At about the same time that I was becoming perplexed over why my patients were not responding to a low-calorie diet, I encountered a patient at the opposite extreme. We'll call him ST.

ST also weighed 170 pounds, the same as LS, the young lady who couldn't lose a pound of fat from a low-calorie diet. But ST wanted to *gain* weight.

His trainer had told him to eat as much protein as possible. But he hadn't gained a pound. When this didn't work, he added more protein. He kept adding more protein until he came to see me. Frustrated, he said, *"Doc I'm up to eating like a pig 6 times a day. I'm stuffed all the time and I can't gain a pound."*

When I looked at his food log, I could hardly believe it. He ate a dozen egg whites a day. He ate 24 ounces of steak at a time, sometimes twice a day. He drank a 40 oz protein shake twice a day. And in between meals, he would scarf down 36 oz of canned tuna and pure protein snacks.

When I totaled the calories, he ate between 4500 and 5000 calories a day for the previous 12 weeks. *And he lost 6 pounds.*

I thought exercise might explain it. But he said, *"No Doc, I'm doing very little. I go to the gym 3 times a week but I don't do cardio and I'm out of there in 20 minutes. I don't want to burn the calories..."*

At first, I thought it must be the difference in the rate these two individuals burn calories at rest. This is called Basal Metabolic Rate (BMR). But to account for such a dramatic difference, the BMR would have to vary by more than 500%.

But research shows only a marginal variation in a person's BMR. Nowhere near that magnitude. Clearly, something else was at play...

What ST had done was discover by accident the most important principal of healthy weight loss. To make weight loss relatively easy and healthy you must over-consume protein.

I mean you must eat more protein than your body is going to use. Why do this? Because this is what throws the metabolic switch. It tells your body that times are good. When times are good, it doesn't need the stored fat. It can now burn that fat for other things.

Fat Loss Myth #2: Eating Fat Makes You Fat

For 30 years, the American Heart Association, the modern food industry and the media have been telling you the secret to fat loss is a low-fat diet. This is a dangerous mistake.

For years, a handful of us in medicine have been telling you the opposite – that dietary fat is not the problem. And when you eat low-fat, you inevitably eat more carbohydrates and inadvertently sacrifice the most important nutrient, protein. This is a prescription for losing vital muscle and turning your body into flab.

All along, we've had a growing body of medical studies backing up our claims. But the governmental organizations have stubbornly clung to their low fat hypothesis and the media has failed to recognize the mounting evidence against it. But over the last few years, that has finally started to change...

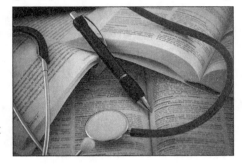

In 2003, *The New York Times Sunday Magazine* ran a cover story entitled "What If It's All Been a Big Fat Lie?" The article said the American medical establishment's worst nightmare had come true – not only had they been wrong about what constitutes a healthy diet, but their recommendations had made the problem worse... and their critics had been right all along.

Let me be clear: eating a low-fat diet not only makes you fatter, but also puts you at risk for a slew of medical problems, from the onset of diabetes to heart disease and stroke.

"As a former long distance runner, I am thrilled with PACE. The sprinting workouts have allowed me to keep running and injury-free. The definition in my muscles and the fact that I am not muscle wasting any more, contributed to an increase in fitness. I now have a better understanding of what it means to be fit. PACE is my cardio program. It requires less time and really delivers. Thank you for sharing this wonderful training program."

Linda O., East Greenwich, RI

Enjoy the Food You Were Designed to Eat

The New York Times Magazine article was largely correct. Hundreds of medical studies have shown that the low fat, high-starch diet advocated by so many has made Americans fatter and sicker.

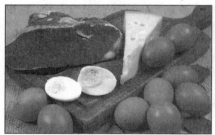

If you want to burn fat, you have to forget about tofu burgers, cereals and whole grain breads. The good news is you can start eating the foods you like. You can eat the things your father probably told you would "put hair on your chest" decades ago – like steak and eggs!

I've helped hundreds of my own patients use this approach. I've seen them make the transformation from fat and sickly to lean and healthy. My clinic is full of patients who used to take multiple medications and now take none. Along with becoming lean, these men and women see their cholesterols and triglycerides drop, their high blood pressures resolve, their pain of arthritis vanish and their diabetes reverse.

Our *Wellness Research Foundation* has collected compelling scientific evidence that not only the modern epidemic of obesity but many "modern" diseases are either caused or worsened by following the diet that you've been told was healthy.

There is still much to be learned about nutrition. But one thing is becoming increasingly clear: The best diet is the diet that we instinctively want to eat. It's the diet we *were* eating – without the help of modern medicine – for eons.

What Did Your Ancient Ancestors Really Have for Dinner?

The earliest evidence of the diet of early man comes from fossils. The record is clear. Early man preferred animal flesh. His whole culture was built around acquiring and consuming meat.

And we can go even further back in time. Man's closest living relative, the chimpanzee, regularly hunts down and consumes animal flesh. The meat is very highly prized with the highest-ranking members consuming their fill first. They show a preference for the fat and the organs of their prey.

When all those vegetarian books were so popular back in the 60s and 70s, primatologists believed most other primates were vegetarians. This was cited as a reason for people to swear off beef and eat bean sprouts instead. I still see this claim being made but we now know it to be false. Most other primates regularly eat insects, forage for small animals and routinely hunt down and eat any game they can kill.

Perhaps even more convincing, is the data from indigenous cultures. Many of these cultures survived unaffected by the modern world into the 20th century. Anthropologists *studied and recorded their dietary habits.*

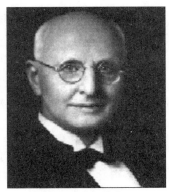

Of particular note is the work of Dr. Weston Price. He traveled throughout the world meticulously documenting their lifestyles. He studied 14 remaining hunter-gatherer cultures.

Weston A. Price
1870 - 1948
Photo © Price-Pottenger
Nutrition Foundation
www.price-pottenger.org

He discovered two very remarkable features in every culture. One, they were universally lean and lacked the modern constellation of diseases. Two, they all prized and ate meat. There was not a single vegetarian culture.

An extensive study of the health of native people was conducted by Dr. Loren Cordain. Dr. Cordain is an expert on primitive dietary habits and a professor of exercise physiology at Colorado State University. He examined the diets of 229 of the world's remaining native societies.

Here's a summary of his findings:

- He also found no vegetarian cultures.
- Game was their principal source of protein and fat.
- Hunted game or fish was highly valued.
- Organ meat was most coveted, often reserved for the privileged.

Dr. Cordain also found hunter-gatherers relied on animal products as their main food source. Animal foods made up 50-65% of the societies' diets. Cordain concluded:

"… this high reliance on animal-based foods coupled with the relatively low carbohydrate content of wild plant foods produces universally characteristic macronutrient consumption ratios in which protein intakes are greater at the expense of carbohydrate." [1]

The fact that native pre-agricultural societies universally ate more protein than the average modern diet surprises my patients. They have read that we eat too much protein.

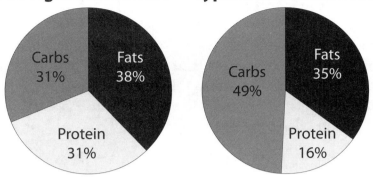

Pre-Agricultural Diet

Carbs 31%
Fats 38%
Protein 31%

Typical American Diet

Carbs 49%
Fats 35%
Protein 16%

The evidence, when taken together, makes one conclusion undeniable: A low-fat vegetarian diet has never been the natural diet of man. The truth is the exact opposite. For millions of years man has eaten meat. What's more, meat was universally prized in every primitive culture.

The Biggest Meat Eaters Don't Get Fat

Politically correct or not, the more meat an indigenous society ate, the healthier it appeared. For instance, the Masai of east Africa who live on raw milk, cattle meat and blood and organ meat appeared to completely lack dental cavities, obesity or heart disease.

Among the healthiest of all native groups studied are the Dinkas. They live along the banks of the Nile River and live mostly on fish and shellfish. One western physician who lived among them reported to have never seen a single case of obesity, heart disease or cancer in 15 years.

"PACE is outstanding. I try to tell everyone I can about it. I even jot down your URL and give it to complete strangers that I meet. Keep up the great work."

Jim W., Plano, TX

Set the Time Machine to 10,000 B.C.
– Back to the Dawn of High Carb Diets

Beginning about 15,000 years ago, some people began to domesticate plants and animals. There was a gradual switch from hunting and gathering to farming. Farming could support a larger population. Quality was traded for quantity. This was the start of the Agricultural Revolution.

Archaeologists can identify the Agricultural Revolution in the fossil record. Human remains tell the tale. But not in the way you might think. Skeletal relics can show the age, gender, height, weight, illnesses, and the state of health of an individual. Archaeologists have found that farming communities were more malnourished and disease ridden than their hunter-gatherer predecessors.

Hunter-gatherer skeletons in Greece show that the average height was about 5'9". Until the advent of agriculture, when Greeks suddenly shrank to a mere 5'. Even today, the Greek population has not fully regained the height of their primitive predecessors.

The record of native people in the Illinois and Ohio River valleys also demonstrate the health consequences of agriculture.

"Archaeologists have excavated some 800 skeletons that paint a picture of the health changes that occurred when a hunter-gatherer culture gave way to the intensive maize farming around A.D. 1150 … these early farmers paid a price for their new-found livelihood. Compared to the hunter-gatherers who proceeded them, the farmers had a nearly 50% increase … in malnutrition, a fourfold increase in iron-deficiency anemia … [and] a threefold rise in infectious disease." [2]

Farmers always grow high-carbohydrate crops. There are no other crops. Even the soybean often touted for is high protein is still over 80% carbohydrate. Other staple crops like potatoes, corn, wheat, and rice are all over 90% carbohydrate.

Farming communities no longer receive the range of nutrients that hunter-gatherers had. And, farmers do not consume high amounts of protein. Malnourished farmers were more susceptible to disease.

The record is consistent. When hunter-gatherers switched to farming, their fat and protein intake went down and their carbohydrate intake went up. The incidence of malnutrition and diseases rose in every case I can find.

Of course, the sudden rise in the modern constellation of diseases did not go unnoticed. In the middle of the last century, it began to be identified as the modern plague.

"Dr. Sears helped me go from a size 16 to a size 10. I am very happy with the way I look now. I actually have a waist! My neighbor hadn't seen me in 3 months and could hardly recognize me. She was amazed and said, 'What on earth have you been doing? You look so good!' For the first time in my life, I'm looking forward to the future."
Theadora W., Wellington, FL

Fat Is Wrongly Blamed for Making People Fat

You can blame a reductionist view of health, you can blame the commercial interest of food producers or slick Madison Avenue marketing but for one reason or another, the cause of the problem was misread.

Without real evidence, fat was identified as the culprit. It was not known that native diets consisted of more fat than modern diets. Endocrinology or the study of hormones was not considered.

If we can divorce ourselves from the prejudice about fat, the endocrinology is really quite simple. Your body controls fat building. Hormones are used to set the controls. The hormone insulin controls fat.

How much insulin do you secrete in response to a fat-laden meal? Zero. Insulin is secreted in response to carbohydrate. Eat more carbohydrate and you will secrete more insulin and build more fat all other things being equal. Fat in the diet, in contrast, is neutral.

Scientists have even recently identified the cellular machinery that turns carbohydrates into fat. Researchers at the University of Texas Southwestern Medical Center found a protein in cells called ChREBP. It converts excess dietary carbohydrates into fat stores.

Big Mistake: Americans Abandon Fat and Go Carb Crazy

In 1977, George McGovern led a Senate Committee that released its "Dietary Goals for the United States." The publication advised that Americans drastically cut their dietary fat intake. And, according to the "Dietary Goals," fat was the cause of illnesses sweeping the nation.

The National Institutes of Health jumped on the "ban fat" wagon. In 1984, NIH announced that Americans must cut their fat intake. In response, the food industry quickly produced a slew of "low fat" products. But without the tasty fat, the food produced was bland. High amounts of sugar became a common additive.

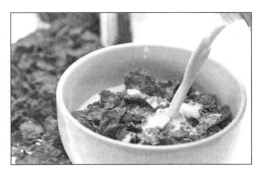

Americans replaced fat with refined carbohydrates and sugar. The amount of calories from fat in the American diet decreased. And, the amount of calories from refined carbohydrates increased… dramatically.

Cereals were cheap to produce and could be sold at a huge profit. When Kellogg and other early proponents of cereals started their health farms, they preached that modern society was oversexed. Eating cereal they claimed would solve the problem.

As bizarre as this and the other inflated and unsubstantiated claims were, there might be a twisted kernel of truth. Cholesterol is the building block for testosterone. If you deprive yourself of animal fat, your testosterone will go down.

Testosterone deficiency has the worst kinds of consequences for men (impotence, depression, obesity and fatigue to name a few). I've seen evidence for this first hand. Some of the most severe testosterone deficiencies I've encountered were in men eating a very low-fat diet. Often, they had gotten this advice from their physicians.

Your Body Needs Essential Fats Every 24 Hours

A huge problem with low fat is that it also means high carb. Excessive intake of carbohydrate is the central dietary problem in my patient population. But there is another problem emerging from the low fat advice: The lower fat intake itself can be detrimental to your health.

One study published in *The American Journal of Clinical Nutrition* found that low-fat diets affect calcium absorption. The study found low-fat diets were associated with 20% lower calcium absorption than higher fat diets.[3]

The American Journal of
CLINICAL NUTRITION

The State University of New York at Buffalo also reported that low-fat diets cause health problems. The researchers found that people who eat low-fat diets develop weaker immune systems.[4]

A certain amount of fat is critical to absorb vitamins. The fat-soluble nutrients like vitamins A, D, E, and K and coenzyme CoQ10 cannot be absorbed without fat.

"I love the PACE. Over the course of about 10 months, I lost 15 lbs. without changing my diet. My body is toned and looks better than it's looked in years. I feel great and love to go to the gym for my 15-20 minute routine. I have great energy and love the way I look. I receive compliments all the time. I even sing better after my routine, which is not an outcome I expected from exercising. I would and do recommend this program all the time. It works, it's simple, takes very little time and has great rewards."

Alison H., Salisbury, MD

Ditch the Modern Diets and Get Back to Your Native Fitness

The good news is that fixing this mess is not as hard as you might think. What was caused by 10-millennia of farming and worsened by weak science and bad advice can be fixed by you alone.

Follow a few simple rules for selecting your food. You will

find a guide to selecting healthy "real natural" foods in this book. You will be able to eat better tasting foods and feel more satisfied. And don't be worried that eating meat is going to drive up your cholesterol.

A number of studies have also been done concerning lean meat and cholesterol. One of the most recent studies has proven that the incorporation of lean meat into the diet helps reduce cholesterol levels. By the way, it didn't matter whether it was white meat and red meat. Both lowered bad LDL cholesterol and raised good HDL cholesterol.[5]

Numerous studies have proven that low-carbohydrate diets improve diabetes. One important study analyzed diabetic patients. The people first ate a low-carb diet with 25% of calories coming from carbohydrates. After 8 weeks, they switched to a high-carb diet with 55% of calories from carbohydrates (very similar to the average American's diet).

During the low-carb diet the people experienced a significant drop in blood sugar levels. When they switched to the high-carb diet they experienced a rise in blood sugar levels and a worsening of their diabetic condition.[6]

The Journal of Nutrition published a German study *JN* THE JOURNAL OF NUTRITION that proved the importance of protein. The researchers found that high-protein diets boost antioxidant levels. The higher the protein consumed, the higher their antioxidant levels became. Low protein consumption actually seemed to induce the oxidative effects of free radicals.[7]

An alarming report out of Stockholm University has raised even more debate about carbohydrates. The report, which was released through Sweden's National Food Administration in April 2002, found cancer-causing agents in breads, rice, potatoes, and cereals. Starch transforms into a compound called acrylamide when heated. Acrylamide is recognized as a carcinogen by the US Environmental Protection Agency.[8]

Burn Fat Faster With This Simple Rule of Thumb

One of your best tools for fat loss is the Glycemic Index (GI). You've probably heard of it. It measures how quickly foods break down into sugar in your bloodstream. High glycemic foods turn into blood sugar very quickly. Starchy foods like potatoes are a good example. Potatoes have such a high GI rating; it's almost the same as eating table sugar.

That's a problem. When your blood sugar levels are up for long periods of time, your body releases a flood of insulin. And all that insulin makes you fat, slow and tired. Remember: insulin tells your body to make and store fat.

I strongly believe in the GI and have been using it for years with amazing results. But, there's a missing piece to it... something that can take you a step further and give you faster, better results. And, it's a tool most people haven't even heard about.

It's called the Glycemic Load (GL).

The GI tells you how fast different foods spike your blood sugar. But the GI won't tell you how much carbohydrate per serving you're getting. That's where the GL is a great help. It measures the amount of carbohydrate in each serving of food.

Why is this important? Some foods are high on the GI. Carrots, for example, rate a 92. But the amount of carbs in one carrot is very low. Carrots rate a 1 on the GL. So even though they are high on the GI, their low GL makes them a good choice.

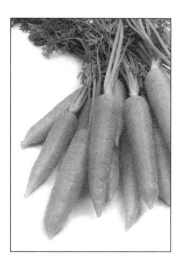

Here's one that may surprise you. Corn rates a 55 on the GI. That's a little high, but would be fine in moderation. Until you look at corn's GL... a whopping 62. That means for every serving of corn you eat, you're getting a huge load of carbohydrate. That makes corn a very fattening food.

Together, the GI and the GL make a powerful duo for helping you make the best food choices possible to shed fat and keep it off.

You Were Born to Eat a Low Glycemic Diet

When your insulin is high, your body becomes less and less responsive to insulin. You then have to secrete more and more insulin to get its job done. It becomes a vicious cycle. And it eventually leads to insulin resistance. Insulin resistance then makes it difficult to regulate blood sugar. You are just asking for diabetes at this point.

The USDA food pyramid recommends that you eat grains, carbs, and starchy foods and it's literally making you sick and fat. But were we born to eat grains?

Farming and grain-based agriculture – the staple of our modern diet – were developed about 10,000 years ago. That's not a very longtime from an evolutionary standpoint.

For millions of years before that, our hunter-gatherer ancestors lived on a diet of meat, wild vegetables, nuts, and berries. Their bodies evolved around a diet that gave them the strength, stamina and muscle growth for the hunt. And genetically speaking, your body is 99.998% identical. As you can see, not much has changed.

Our ancestors did something right. They followed a low-glycemic diet. Lean meats, nuts, berries… all low glycemic. They developed this diet all on their own without books or charts. There was no science behind it. It was all they knew. And it kept them lean and healthy.

Follow the Glycemic "Speed Limit" for Faster Fat Loss

Different kinds of carbs have different effects on your body. All digestible carbs are converted to glucose in the bloodstream eventually, but how rapidly that conversion takes place and how long the resulting increase in blood sugar lasts makes a huge difference to your health.

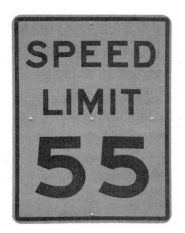

Many people think sweet foods have a greater impact on blood sugar, but natural simple sugars like those found in honey and fruit tend to be much easier on the body's glucose/insulin balance than complex starchy foods like breads, breakfast cereals and potatoes. The complex starches create a rapid glucose reaction in your body, while the simple sugars don't have the same negative effect.

The GI is what we use to measure how rapidly carbs in a food convert to sugar in your bloodstream compared to straight glucose. The higher the glycemic index, the higher the spike in blood sugar the food will cause.

Spikes in blood sugar create an excessive insulin response. Foods with a low GI contain carbs that break down slowly and release smaller, more manageable amounts of glucose into your bloodstream.

Keep this in mind: foods with a GI of 60 or above are high; those between 0 and 40 are low. Foods in the middle should be eaten in moderation. Here at my clinic, I tell my patients to eat below 40.

Like the GI, high GL foods have a greater impact on blood sugar. A GL above 20 is high. Below 10 is low. Foods in the middle range are medium.

> "PACE has helped my husband to lower his diabetic medications, and our goal is to have him off all medications within the year."
>
> Diane Z., New York City, NY

Foods with a glycemic load under 10 are good choices – these foods should be your first choice for carbs. Foods that fall between 10 and 20 on the glycemic load scale have a moderate effect on your blood sugar. Foods with a glycemic load above 20 will cause blood sugar and insulin spikes – eat these foods sparingly.

Different tables of glycemic load will vary because they may use different serving sizes. In the table beginning on page 193, I've included a GL value that reflects a realistic serving size – the serving sizes of foods are also included. You may notice when you look at the chart that meats aren't included. Meat is carb free so it doesn't affect blood sugar.

Follow the Numbers to Your Ideal Body Composition

A food may have a high GI ranking because of the way its carbs convert to sugar, but the actual amount of carbs in the food may be so low that the overall effect isn't so bad.

When making food choices, you need to consider both GI and GL because GI alone can sometimes be misleading. Remember the carrot? Here's another: Watermelon has a high GI rank of 72. Judging by GI alone, it would be a poor food choice. But its GL is very low, so while its carbs convert very quickly into sugar, there isn't much for your body to contend with. The overall effect on blood sugar is very moderate.

On the other hand, white rice seems okay when you just look at GI. Most brands of white rice have a GI of around 50. But they have a high GL, so even though the carbs in the rice may not convert as fast, there's a lot of carbs there for your body to deal with. Pasta is another example. Spaghetti ranks a medium level GI, but its GL is very high, making it fattening if you eat it often.

Ice cream, which also has a fairly high GI of about 60 has a very low glycemic load – just a 6! That means the amount of carbs you're getting from ice cream is small, despite the sugar. If you want to indulge, ice cream is a safe bet, but in moderation.

Here's another surprise… One ounce of a Dove dark chocolate bar has a low GI of 23 and a low GL of about 4. Who doesn't like chocolate? So enjoy this one too.

There are many other foods that you may think of as sweet, and therefore off limits – like fruit. Cantaloupe has a high GI of 65 so you might think it's off limits, but it has a low GL of 7.8. So, again, you are only getting a small amount of carbs regardless of the sugar content. So try some sweet cantaloupe for a treat.

Simple sugars in moderation are fine – complex carbohydrates or starches are more of a problem. For example, you might think that because it's not sweet a piece of corn bread would have a low GI, but think again. It has a whopping 110 GI and almost a 31 GL. This one will spike your blood sugar through the roof. This is one you want to avoid.

Below is a chart I put together combining both glycemic index and glycemic load numbers for some favorite foods. I use this chart with my own patients.

When using this chart a good rule of thumb is to stick to foods with a GI of 40 or below and a GL of 10 or below. Stick to those numbers and you'll see results.

Food	Glycemic Index	Serving Size	Glycemic Load
CANDY/SWEETS			
Honey	87	2 tbsp	17.9
Jelly Beans	78	1 oz	22
Snickers Bar	68	60g (1/2 bar)	23
Table Sugar	68	2 tsp	7
Strawberry Jam	51	2 tbsp	10.1
Peanut M&M's	33	30g (1 oz)	5.6
Dove Dark Chocolate Bar	23	37g (1 oz)	4.4

BAKED GOODS & CEREALS			
Angel food cake	67	28g (1 slice)	10.7

Food	Glycemic Index	Serving Size	Glycemic Load
Bagel	72	89g (1/4 in.)	33
Blueberry Muffin	59	113g (1 med)	30
Bran Flakes	74	29g (3/4 cup)	13.3
Bran Muffin	60	113g (1 med)	30
Cheerios	74	30g (1 cup)	13.3
Chocolate cake w/ chocolate frosting	38	64g (1 slice)	12.5
Corn Bread	110	60g (1 piece)	30.8
Corn Chex	83	30g (1 cup)	20.8
Corn Flakes	92	28g (1 cup)	21.1
Corn pops	80	31g (1 cup)	22.4
Corn tortilla	70	24g (1 tortilla)	7.7
Croissant, Butter	67	57g (1 med)	17.5
Donut (large glazed)	76	75g (1 donut)	24.3
French Bread	95	64g (1 slice)	29.5
Graham Cracker	74	14g (2 sqrs)	8.1
Grape Nuts	75	58g (1/2 cup)	31.5
Kaiser Roll	73	57g (1 roll)	21.2
Kellogg's Special K	69	31g (1 cup)	14.5
Melba Toast	70	12g (4 rounds)	5.6
Muselix	66	55g (2/3 cup)	23.8
Oatmeal	58	117g (1/2 cup)	6.4
Oatmeal Cookie	55	18g (1 large)	6
Oatmeal, Instant	65	234g (1 cup)	13.7
Popcorn	55	8g (1 cup)	2.8
Pound cake, Sara Lee	54	30g (1 piece)	8.1
Pumpernickel bread	41	26g (1 slice)	4.5

Food	Glycemic Index	Serving Size	Glycemic Load
Raisin Bran	61	61g (1 cup)	24.4
Rice Krispies	82	33g (1.25 cup)	23
Rye bread, 100% whole	65	32g (1 slice)	8.5
Rye Krisp Crackers	65	25 (1 wafer)	11.1
Taco Shell	68	13g (1 med)	4.8
Vanilla Cake and Vanilla Frosting	42	64g (1 slice)	16
Waffle (homemade)	76	75g (1 waffle)	18.7
Wheat Bread	70	28g (1 slice)	7.7
White Bread	70	25g (1 slice)	8.4
Whole wheat pita	57	64g (1 pita)	17

BEVERAGES			
Apple Juice	41	248g (1 cup)	11.9
Cola, Carbonated	63	370g (12oz can)	25.2
Cranberry Juice Cocktail	68	253g (1 cup)	24.5
Gatorade Powder	78	16g (.75 scoop)	11.7
Grapefruit Juice, sweetened	48	250g (1 cup)	13.4
Hot Chocolate Mix	51	28g (1 packet)	11.7
Orange Juice	57	249g (1 cup)	14.25
Pineapple Juice	46	250g (1 cup)	14.7
Soy Milk	44	245g (1 cup)	4
Tomato Juice	38	243g (1 cup)	3.4

DAIRY			
Ice Cream (Lower Fat)	47	76g (1/2 cup)	9.4

Food	Glycemic Index	Serving Size	Glycemic Load
Ice Cream	38	72g (1/2 cup)	6
Milk, Whole	40	244g (1 cup)	4.4
Pudding	44	100g (1/2 cup)	8.4
Yogurt, Plain	36	245g (1 cup)	6.1

LEGUMES

Food	Glycemic Index	Serving Size	Glycemic Load
Baked Beans	48	253g (1 cup)	18.2
Chickpeas, Boiled	31	240g (1 cup)	13.3
Kidney Beans	27	256g (1 cup)	7
Lentils	29	198g (1 cup)	7
Lima Beans	31	241g (1 cup)	7.4
Peanuts	13	146g (1 cup)	1.6
Pinto Beans	39	171g (1 cup)	11.7
Soy Beans	20	172g (1 cup)	1.4

VEGETABLES

Food	Glycemic Index	Serving Size	Glycemic Load
Beets, canned	64	246g (1/2 cup)	9.6
Broccoli, cooked	0	78g (1/2 cup)	0
Cabbage, cooked	0	75g (1/2 cup)	0
Carrot, raw	92	15g (1 large)	1
Celery, raw	0	62g (1 stalk)	0
Corn, yellow	55	166g (1 cup)	61.5
Cauliflower	0	100g (1 cup)	0
Green Beans	0	135g (1 cup)	0
Mushrooms	0	70g (1 cup)	0
Parsnip	97	78g (1/2 cup)	11.6
Peas, Frozen	48	72g (1/2 cup)	3.4

Food	Glycemic Index	Serving Size	Glycemic Load
Potato	104	213g (1 med)	36.4
Spinach	0	30g (1 cup)	0
Sweet Potato	54	133g (1 cup)	12.4
Tomato	38	123g (1 med)	1.5
Yam	51	136g (1 cup)	16.8

FRUIT			
Apples, w/ skin	39	138g (1 med)	6.2
Apricot, canned in light syrup	64	253g (1 cup)	24.3
Apricot, dried	32	130g (1 cup)	23
Banana	51	118g (1 med)	12.2
Cantaloupe	65	177g (1 cup)	7.8
Fruit Cocktail, drained	55	214g (1 cup)	19.8
Grapes	43	92g (1 cup)	6.5
Grapefruit	25	123g (1/2 fruit)	2.8
Kiwi, w/ skin	58	76g (1 fruit)	5.2
Mango	51	165g (1 cup)	12.8
Orange	48	140g (1 fruit)	7.2
Papaya	60	140g (1 cup)	6.6
Peach	28	98g (1 med)	2.2
Peaches, canned, heavy syrup	58	262g (1 cup)	28.4
Peaches, canned, light syrup	52	251g (1 cup)	17.7
Pears	33	166g (1 med)	6.9
Pears, canned in pear juice	44	248g (1 cup)	12.3

Food	Glycemic Index	Serving Size	Glycemic Load
Pineapple, raw	66	155g (1 cup)	11.9
Plum	24	66g (1 fruit)	1.7
Prunes	29	132g (1 cup)	34.2
Raisins	64	43g (small box)	20.5
Strawberries	40	152g (1 cup)	3.6
Sweet Cherries, raw	22	117g (1 cup)	3.7
Watermelon	72	152g (1 cup)	7.2

Now that you know how to use the glycemic index and glycemic load here are some easy guidelines to help you build meals that are nutritious and burn fat:

- Choose vegetables that are low-glycemic. These are typically vegetables that grow above the ground like cabbage, broccoli, cauliflower, and asparagus. Other low-glycemic vegetables like mushrooms, green beans, leafy green vegetables, and tomatoes also make good choices. Eat 3 to 5 servings per day.

- For fruits, choose berries and fruits you can eat with the skin on. Eat 1 to 2 servings per day. Avoid dried fruits and fruit juices.

- Eat a high-protein breakfast every morning. This will stabilize your blood sugar and get you off to a good start.

- Avoid grains, including corn.

- Avoid potatoes and foods made with potatoes. Avoid other white foods, like white rice, sugar, and salt.

- All meats, fish and poultry are the real "guilt-free" foods. A good old-fashioned steak won't raise your blood sugar and the protein will help you handle insulin better, build muscle and repair tissue – all essential for staying lean and preventing diabetes.

- Eat grass-fed beef, free-range poultry, wild-caught fish and cage-free eggs to avoid the environmental toxins, hormones and antibiotics. Pick fish that is high in Omega-3s like wild salmon.

- Try making protein the focus of each meal. It kicks your metabolism into high gear.

- Snack on nuts and seeds. They are a good protein source and have Omega 3s. And they keep you full. Have 1 to 2 servings a day.

- Avoid processed foods. They are loaded with bad carbs, artificial sweeteners, and preservatives.

- Avoid trans fats – pick foods with no partially or fully hydrogenated oils. Get healthy fat from lean proteins (grass-fed beef), wild fish, olives/olive oil, avocados, and nuts.

- Avoid high-fructose corn syrup (HFCS). It contributes to insulin resistance. More fructose is converted to fat than other sweeteners – in fact, HFCS has been conclusively linked to obesity. Limit natural sweeteners like sugar and honey.

Endnotes

1 Cordain L, Miller JB, Eaton SB, Mann N, Holt SH, Speth JD. Plant-animal subsistence ratios and macronutrient energy estimations in worldwide hunter-gatherer diets. *Am J Clin Nutr.* 2000; 71(3): 682-692.

2 Diamond J. The Worst Mistake in the Human Race. *Discover Magazine.* May 1987: 64-66.

3 Wolf RL, Cauley JA, Baker CE, et al. Factors associated with calcium absorption efficiency in pre- and perimenopausal women. *Am J Clin Nutr.* 2000;72(2): 466-471.

4 Venkatraman JT, Leddy J, Pendergast D. Dietary fats and immune status in athletes: clinical implications. *Med Sci Sports Exer.* 2000 Jul;32(7Suppl):S389-395.

5 Hunninghake DB, Maki KC, Kwiterovich PO Jr, Davidson MH, Dicklin MR, Kafonek SD. Incorporation of Lean Red Meat into a National Cholesterol Education Program Step I Diet: A Long-Term, Randomized Clinical Trial in Free-Living Persons with Hypercholesterolemia. *J Am Coll Nutr.* 2000;19(3): 351-360.

6 Gutierrez M, Akhavan M, Jovanovic L, Peterson CM. Utility of a Short-Term 25% Carbohydrate Diet on Improving Glycemic Control in Type 2 Diabetes Mellitus. *J Am Coll Nutr.* 1998;17(6):595-600.

7 Petzke KJ, Elsner A, Proll J, Thielecke F, Metges CC. Long-Term High Protein Intake Does Not Increase Oxidative Stress in Rats. *J Nutr.* 2000;130(12): 2889-2896.

8 Törnqvist M. Acrylamide in food: the discovery and its implications: a historical perspective. *Adv Exp Med Biol.* 2005;561:1-19.

PATIENT STORY

Steve McGuire

Steve is one of the most dramatic successes I've seen with PACE during my research. At one point he lost 67 pounds of fat over an 8-week stretch. Overall, Steve:

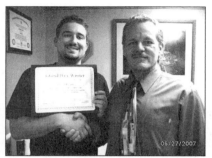

Steve won my PACE fat-loss challenge after losing 88 pounds.

- Lost 88 pounds of fat in 7 months
- Built 42 pounds of new muscle
- Brought his body fat percentage from 50% all the way down to 17.1%
- Lowered his triglycerides (blood fat) from 370 to 177

When Steve came to see me he said his biggest problem was losing weight and keeping it off. Again, PACE provided big gains in record time. You can see the dramatic changes from his records:

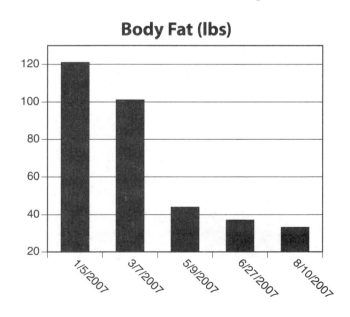

Body Fat (lbs)

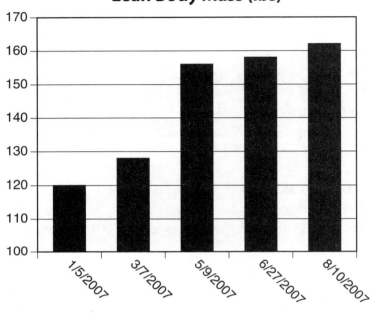

Lean Body Mass (lbs)

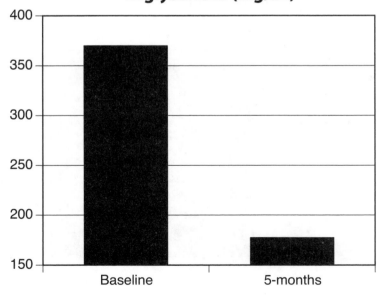

Triglycerides (mg/dL)

CHAPTER ELEVEN

Pocket-Sized PACE Power

You don't need a gym or special equipment to practice PACE. But there are nutrients that can help improve your performance. Some keep you lean, some give you energy when you need it, others help your blood vessels expand, ramping up oxygen delivery.

In this chapter I'll show you why they work and how to use them. They're safe, effective and inexpensive. Best of all, they keep you feeling great.

Give Your Body Power for High Performance

What do I mean by power?

It's strength and energy. It's the ability to keep working. It's having both the muscle and the mind to get things done.

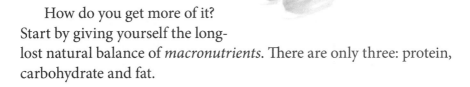

How do you get more of it? Start by giving yourself the long-lost natural balance of *macronutrients*. There are only three: protein, carbohydrate and fat.

Get them in the right combination and you give yourself the right hormonal signal for power on demand – whenever you need it. And there's more: this winning formula helps you slim down too.

Let me explain how it works.

Use This Caveman Secret for Real Power and Super Strength

Your ancient ancestors never had a problem picking the right nutrients. And they never got tired or fat doing it. They had everything in the right balance: an abundance of lean protein, healthy carbs in low doses and lots of good fats.

In today's world it's a lot harder. If you're like most Americans, you're not getting the balance you need to stay active, alert, and on the move.

> *"Dr. Sears, thank you for all of your great work. I've lost 6 lbs. in 2 weeks with PACE."*
> Tom P., Maryland Heights, MO

It's easy to fall short on protein, load up on carbs and get all the wrong fats. And when you look for something to keep you going, it's usually full of sugar or empty carbs.

Extra protein will help you slim down and pack on pounds of new muscle. Remember, extra protein tells your body "times are good." It gives your body the feeling that you have an abundant source of good food. In response, your body burns fat as fuel.

But there's more to the story… extra protein is a good idea, but when you combine it with low carbs and good fats, you'll get usable energy that pumps up your muscles and the brain food that keeps your mind sharp and clear – all in one tasty super food.

Good fats – like omega-3s – power up your brain. Your brain is more than 60% fat, and it needs a regular supply of good fats to keep it fired up. The power bar I designed has a potent complex of omega-3s with a shot of coconut oil, one of healthiest oils for your heart and brain.

Having the right carbs is critical. Eat too much of the wrong kind and you'll wind up feeling slow and tired. And you'll get fat too... but keep a tight rein on your blood sugar and you'll get all the energy you need without putting on any extra fat.

I've applied these same principles to help you eat between meals without weight gain or a loss of energy. They also work well right after a PACE workout, as they provide a reliable source of muscle-building protein that won't spike your blood sugar.

When you're shopping for your own power bars, make sure they're free of artificial sweeteners, grains and/or empty carbs. They won't give you the results you want. Put the focus on protein and natural, low-glycemic ingredients.

Finally... Snack Food Without the Guilt or Guesswork

When I put patients on my PACE program, I always monitor their diet. And I often recommend they eat five or six smaller meals a day instead of two or three big ones.

That means healthy snacking is an integral part of your PACE program.

Snack foods are a little different than the power bars mentioned above. A power bar should give you a good shot of protein and healthy carbs to prepare you for a workout or help you recover afterward. Snack foods can be more varied in their ingredients as long as they maintain the right blend of macronutrients.

So how do you shop for the right snack foods? Even if you go for one of those "health food bars" you'll be surprised when you read the label. They're often packed with all kinds of stuff that makes you feel fat and bloated.

Here's the problem: the manufacturer doesn't know what's supposed to be in it. They fill their products full of sugar and artificial ingredients, or they decide to go "natural" and stuff them with bird food and fake sweeteners. Either way, you lose.

Leave the Bird Food for the Birds...

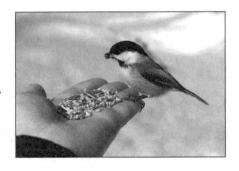

One of the biggest "junk science" myths is the notion that you need "healthy grains" to be healthy. What do these experts consider healthy grains? Wheat... Soy... Corn... Oats... all the vegetarian garbage that's no better than bird food.

Here's a little surprise: *there are no healthy grains*. And no matter what they try and tell you, these grains are never low on the glycemic index.

Corn is one of the worst offenders. And these days, it's in everything. It's one of the big food makers' favorite fillers. In some forms, corn has a GI rating of over 100! (That's at the top of the scale.)

Leave bird food for the birds. Your body doesn't need corn and wheat. It will only make you fat and tired. Even if it's part of a so-called healthy snack.

The companies that make most snack foods think this stuff is good for you. They put "made with soy" on their label like it's some kind of badge of honor. Little do they know that soy is highly estrogenic. Eat enough of it, and it actually *increases* your risk of some forms of cancer. Never mind that it makes you fat.

> *"I'm a 53-year-old ex-sporting fanatic who had 'let it all go' since ceasing real sports about 15 years ago.*
>
> *I started PACE – treadmill, stepper, rowing, cycling and, Hindu squats. My exercising heart rate has improved as well as my recovery times. I never get on the scales anymore, but my jeans tell me what I need to know – down from a 38-inch to a 32-inch waist.*
>
> *PACE has changed not only my physical life but my outlook and self-esteem – many, many thanks."*
>
> Steve M., Exeter, United Kingdom

Avoid the Stuff That's Sickly Sweet

Another pitfall in most snack foods is the way they sweeten it. Think about this for a moment… if you eat a "health bar" that's full of corn, soy and wheat, do you think it's going to taste good? Of course not. Without any sweetener, they would taste like sandpaper.

To hide the fact that what they're giving you is little more than pulverized bird food, they inject a shot of *high fructose corn syrup* (HFCS) to keep you from throwing it back up. Seriously, HFCS is not even a natural product. The enzymes they use to turn corn into a sweetener are genetically modified. You'd never find this stuff in nature.

Even worse, it wreaks havoc on your body. First, it cuts off a critical hormone called *leptin*. This is the messenger that tells your brain that your stomach is full. Without it, you keep eating and eating. Second, it has a very high GI rating and floods your blood with a tidal wave of sugar. Clinical studies link HFCS to obesity, diabetes, metabolic syndrome and a higher risk of heart disease.

You don't need this junk either. You can eat naturally sweet without any of the problems or side effects. Most fruits have a low GI rating and give you great taste without the extra fat around your waist.

Get Real Energy From Fat

A lot of my patients look at me funny when I tell them they can get real energy from fat. They're so conditioned to think that fat is bad, they have a hard time believing the reality: Good fat is good for you.

What's more, good fat will give you a boost of energy and make you feel like you've really eaten something – not that hollow feeling you get from eating grains.

One of the easiest to get in a real snack food is ALA. This is a kind of omega-3 fatty acid that helps your body burn fat as energy. That means the fat in your blood stream is much less likely to be stored as fat. It's a win-win situation. You get an extra boost of energy, and your body gets rid of fat that otherwise would have landed around your waist.

Your other best source of energy comes from protein. This is the number one ingredient that's missing in most "energy on the go" foods. Your body needs good protein sources to create ATP – your body's fastest, most usable energy source.

ATP (adenosine triphosphate) is the stuff your body burns first when you ask it to do something. Ever wonder why you can only sprint for a minute or two at a time? ATP is the answer. It's high-power energy, but you only have small amounts of it. Good protein helps put it back.

Put a Bulletproof Vest Around Your Immune System

Antioxidants are critical to good health and they should be a part of the foods you eat every day. Antioxidants protect every cell, tissue and organ in your body – keeping them healthier, longer.

It's just like a sandwich. If you leave it on the counter, the air makes the bread stale. And if you leave it out for a few days, the meat and cheese go rotten. (This destructive process is called *oxidation*. Oxidation is carried out by *free radicals*.)

But seal it in a Ziploc bag and throw it in the fridge, and it stays good for weeks. Your body is the same. Give your cells the right antioxidant protection and your body will last years – even decades – longer.

All-Natural "Primal Snack"
– a Real PACE Partner

I combined some of the healthiest nuts and seeds, all packed with protein and healthy fats. In spite of the variety, the flavor is simple and light. Add to that some of the best antioxidant fruits like cranberries and blueberries and you've got a real fast food that's high in energy – without any of the junk.

- **Almonds:** Helps lower LDL "bad cholesterol" and provides a great source of protein, vitamin E, magnesium and potassium. Rich in powerful antioxidants called phytochemicals.

- **Sunflower Seeds:** High in folate (B9), healthy fats, vitamin E, selenium and copper. Rich in powerful antioxidants called phytochemicals.

- **Flax Seeds:** Powerful healthy fats that normalize cholesterol, triglycerides and blood pressure. One of the best plant sources of brain-boosting omega-3 fatty acids.

- **Currants:** Renowned for vitamin C (a powerful antioxidant), GLA (Gamma-Linoleic Acid, a very rare essential fatty acid) and potassium. They have four times the vitamin C of oranges, and twice the antioxidants of blueberries.

- **Cranberries:** Powerful source of antioxidants called phenols. Research shows that cranberries can reduce LDL (bad) cholesterol levels and raise levels of HDL (good) cholesterol in the blood.

- **Cashews:** Great source of protein and healthy fats with high levels of the essential minerals iron, magnesium, phosphorus, zinc, copper and manganese.

- **Pumpkin Seeds:** One of nature's most powerful seeds.

Protects your prostate, lowers LDL (bad) cholesterol, lowers your risk of osteoporosis (brittle bones) and provides a great source of heart-healthy magnesium.

- **Blueberries:** Ranked number one in antioxidants when compared to 40 other fruits, blueberries are packed with tannins and anthocyanins that have been linked to prevention and even reversal of age-related mental decline.

- **Coconut Oil:** Easily the healthiest oil you can eat. It is rich in lauric acid, which is known for being antiviral, antibacterial and antifungal, and contains zero trans fats. Promotes heart health, fat loss and youthful skin.

Fuel Your PACE Program With Nature's Most Powerful Nutrient: Protein

In ancient times our ancestors thrived on a diet high in protein. It kept their hearts strong and allowed for consistent new muscle growth. In today's world we're taught that somehow protein is bad... that if we eat too much we'll get sick.

Nothing could be further from the truth. Good protein sources give you the essential amino acids your body needs every 24 hours. These amino acids are called "essential" because our body can't make them on its own. They need to come from your diet.

> "At 53, my level of fitness and flexibility marvels my physician at the VA and my friends and family. I applaud your efforts in getting people to exercise scientifically and with realistic goals."
>
> Jose A., Altamonte Springs, FL

For your PACE program to be successful, you need to fuel it with the right kind of energy. Over consuming protein keeps you lean and muscular. Your body depends on it; especially after exercise.

University Study Reveals:
Protein After a Workout Builds New Muscle

Researchers at McMaster University in Canada tested three different supplement drinks after exercise.

Six men finished a two-hour stationary bike ride on three separate occasions. After one trial they drank a carb-only drink. (Providing 1.2 g of carbohydrate per kg of body weight.)

After another trial they drank a protein-carb drink. (Providing the same amount of carbohydrate plus 0.4 g of protein per kg of body weight.)

And after the third trial they drank another carb-only drink. (Providing as many total calories as the carb-protein drink but without any protein.)

The researchers found that the carb-protein trial resulted in a higher rate of protein synthesis than the two carb-only trials. Only in the carb-protein trial was the whole-body net protein balance positive.

That means there was muscle gain only in the protein group, and a net muscle loss when the carb-only drinks were consumed. The study was published in the *Journal of Applied Physiology*.

Rasmussen BB, Tipton KD, Miller SL, Wolf SE, Wolfe RR. An oral essential amino acid-carbohydrate supplement enhances muscle protein anabolism after resistance exercise. *J Appl Physiol*, 2000; 88(2): 386 - 392.

A landmark study published in the *Journal of Applied Physiology* found that a supplement of protein and carbs consumed within an hour to three hours after intense exertion increased muscle synthesis.[1]

That means a protein supplement after PACE triggers new muscle growth.

Interestingly, the same study showed that a carb-only drink consumed after intense exertion resulted in a net muscle loss. So skip the Gatorade and stick to high-protein drinks and supplements that include low-glycemic carbs.

Here are a few reliable ways to get more protein into your workout and daily routine.

Raw Eggs: The Perfect Super Food

Many experts in the field of nutrition are finally waking up to what athletes, body builders and long-lived people already know. Some raw foods offer far more and better nutrients. Case in point: eggs.

You probably don't relish the idea of guzzling raw eggs. But there is good reason to. Raw eggs offer something that cooked eggs can't. It's much easier than you might think. I do it everyday.

Eggs may be the only *100% complete food*. They have all the vitamins and minerals you need. They are

| Eggs: Nature's Perfect Protein ||
Food Source	Protein Rating
Eggs	*100*
Fish	70
Beef	69
Milk	60
Nuts	48
Soybeans	47
Whole Wheat	44
Beans	34
Potatoes	34

the only protein source with a quality rating of 100 because they have every amino acid you need in exactly the ratios you need.

Eggs are the highest quality protein you can eat, cooked or raw. However, you'll absorb a raw egg in as little as 30 minutes, where it takes 2 to 4 hours to digest cooked eggs.

Raw eggs are an excellent source of the essential fatty acid, DHA. Docosahexaenoic acid or DHA can ease:[2]

- Hypertension
- Depression
- Brain function
- Heart disease
- Arthritis
- Diabetes
- Cancer

But there's more to the story: It seems the cooking process may reduce other nutrients in your eggs. Cooking eggs denatures their DHA. Along with DHA, other nutrients and proteins collapse in the cooking process.

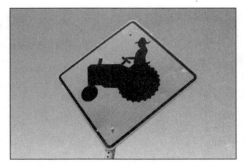

Raw eggs are safe to eat. I've done it myself and recommended it for 30 years. Some people are afraid of salmonella bacteria. But I've never seen a case from modernly produced eggs and the US Department of Agriculture estimates that 0.00003% of eggs in the US have salmonella.[3] That's a very tiny percentage. But still, I recommend locally farmed organic eggs and washing the eggs well before cracking.

Adding raw eggs to your diet is very easy to do. The simplest way is to add a raw egg to a protein shake in the morning. If you are a little hesitant, add a small amount of the egg the first few days, then progressively add more as you get more comfortable.

You can also just drink the egg. This is the quickest way. My father liked to punch a hole in the eggshell and suck it dry. I prefer to crack them into a glass of water, stir and gulp it down. They have no flavor when they're fresh, but the texture may be a little intimidating at first. Just think of it as an oyster. Eat one or two eggs each day to ensure a healthy brain and heart and boost your athletic performance.

There are a few things you should look for before you eat any raw egg:

- Cage-free, no-hormone eggs are best.
- Don't eat the egg if the shell is cracked.
- Only eat eggs that roll "wobbly."
- Do not eat the egg if it smells at all.
- Only eat eggs that have a gel-like white and a firm, round yolk.

Protein: How Much Do You Really Need?

The importance of protein can be summed up in one word: *nitrogen*. Nitrogen is responsible for creating every muscle in your body and fueling cellular regeneration. And the only source of nitrogen you have is protein.

For every 50 grams of protein you'll get 8 grams of nitrogen. To put it in perspective, your heart alone requires 8 grams of nitrogen a day to function normally.[4] So imagine eating only 40 to 60 grams of protein a day like many diets recommend? It's no wonder your muscles grow weak over time and as you age.

Quality protein should be the focal point of every meal. Try to eat one gram of protein for every pound of lean body tissue a day. So if you're a 180-lb. man with 15% body fat you have 153 lbs. of lean muscle mass. That means you should eat 153 grams of protein each day. (To find your lean body mass, refer back to Chapter 7.)

To improve your protein intake you should be eating steak, eggs, chicken, turkey and lots of fish. Fish has a complete mixture of all essential amino acids in a bio-available, rapidly absorbable protein.

Wild-caught fish is low in unhealthy fats and high in omega-3 fatty acids, which keep your heart and brain healthy. (And when it comes to beef, choose grass-fed beef if you can. It's a bit more expensive, but it's packed with healthy omega-3s.)

Counting grams of protein is easy. Here's a quick guide to the most common foods:[5]

How Much Protein Are You Getting? Protein From Animal Sources		
Food Source	Portion Size	Grams of Protein
Beef steak, lean	3 oz	26 grams
Ground beef, lean	3 oz	21 grams
Poultry	3 oz	21 grams
Fish (salmon, trout)	3 oz	21 grams
Pork chop, lean	3 oz	20 grams
Cottage cheese	½ cup	14 grams
Yogurt	1 cup	12 grams
Milk	1 cup	9 grams
Hard cheeses, (cheddar, etc.)	1 oz	7 grams
Egg	1 large	7 grams

There are plant sources of protein but you'll make a sacrifice in terms of quality. None of them are close to having the perfect balance you find in eggs. And many – like rice and bread – are starchy and high on the glycemic index.[6]

How Much Protein Are You Getting? Protein From Plant Sources		
Food Source	**Portion Size**	**Grams of Protein**
Nuts (cashews)	1 cup	21 grams
Tofu	4 oz	9 grams
Legumes, cooked	½ cup	8 grams
Cereals	1 cup	2 to 6 grams
Peanut Butter	1 tbsp	4 grams
Rice	½ cup	3 grams
Pasta	1 cup	3 grams
Seeds	2 tbsp	3 grams
Vegetables	½ cup	2 grams
Bread	1 slice	2 grams

Start keeping track of your protein intake on a daily basis. You'll be amazed how much better you feel. And if you're not getting enough protein from your diet, make sure you take a protein supplement.

Ramp Up Your Athletic Performance With Better Blood Flow

There's an aspect of your PACE program that's linked to your heart, blood vessels, muscle mass and sexual capacity.

I'm talking about *potency.*

Potency is a combination of strength, desire, muscle mass and readiness for sex. It's a feeling of extraordinary potential, like having your foot on the accelerator of a turbo-charged exotic.

Potency is power on demand; whether you're working out or simply getting out of bed. And it's a term that applies to women too.

In medical terms potency is all about *blood flow*. That means getting oxygen-rich blood to every part of your body at a moment's notice. It's easy for young people because their veins and arteries easily expand to handle the extra flow.

As you get older, your veins and arteries get narrow and stiff. But you can restore youthful blood flow at any age.

And you'll get back all the luxuries that come with it.

These include:

- Bigger, harder and more frequent erections. (Better, more intense sexual response for women.)
- Surging waves of desire and arousal.
- Pumping, well-defined muscles.
- Increased stamina, strength and mobility.

Use the Power of Viagra Without Taking the Drug

The secret to big blood flow is nitric oxide, (NO). It's the chemical from the lining of your blood vessels that makes them expand.

Most people think of blood vessels as rigid tubes. Kind of like the pipes in your house. But blood vessels are like balloons. They expand and contract rapidly. When they're open full-throttle they can move tremendous amounts of blood. But when they're too narrow you're in big trouble.

Here's the real problem: As you get older, your supply of NO drops off. Your body just doesn't make as much as it used to. That makes it much harder for your arteries to expand. And if your blood vessels can't expand, blood can't get into your penis. That means no erection and no sex. For women, a lack of blood flow deadens the sexual experience and limits arousal.

> *"I started PACE about a week ago and am very impressed with it. Bottom line is it makes sense and I'm already seeing results."*
>
> Joe S., Greer, SC

This is similar to how Viagra works. Viagra binds to the enzymes that destroy NO. By knocking out the stuff that gets rid of NO your body has the chance to accumulate more of it. As soon as that happens – usually 30 to 40 minutes after taking the pill – you're in business.

As far as drugs go, Viagra isn't a bad one. But its effects diminish over time. The studies I've seen show that over 50% of men stop using Viagra after three years because it stopped working.

There is good news though… by giving your body a particular nutrient, you can get your body to create more NO. As much as you can handle. This breakthrough is not a substitute for Viagra, but works in a similar way. And it's not a drug.

As you'll see, getting more NO does a lot more than give you big, hard erections or better sexual response. All that extra blood flow brings back the thing that really matters: potency.

Potency grows your muscles, makes your heart a tireless warrior and brings the desire back to your bedroom life.

Does Your Whole Body
Have Erectile Dysfunction?

Potency is about blood flow. When you don't have it, major systems in your body start to shut down. The "big three" are:

- Muscle strength
- Sexual performance
- Heart health

Breakdown in these critical areas gives you a kind of *whole body erectile dysfunction*.

You can improve all three areas by practicing PACE. By boosting your blood flow, your body is more apt to make the adaptive responses that improve heart health, new muscle growth and bedroom performance.

Your blood vessels need NO to help them expand. Every vein, artery and capillary – a network that spans thousands of miles – is dependent on NO for survival. Without NO, life would not be possible.

Your heart is a good example. Without NO your heart has to work overtime to move blood through your body. Over time, even the major arteries that lead into and out of the four chambers of your heart will start to harden. Of course, this dramatically increases your chance of heart attack.

And that's just for starters. When your blood vessels are stiff, your major organs don't get the oxygen they need. And that wipes out your energy supply. Your muscles suffer too. Without blood and oxygen, your muscles shrink and start to atrophy.

Your sex life is next on the list. When your blood supply is weak and slow, there's no way to get a good, solid erection. You've probably seen articles in the news showing the connection between erectile dysfunction and heart disease. That's why.

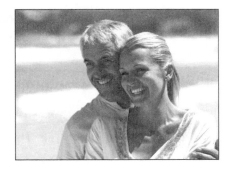

Viagra Started Off As a Heart Drug

Viagra was originally tested as a heart drug. Researchers were looking for a way to improve blood flow by tinkering with NO. And they were successful, but not in the way they intended.

Instead of helping heart patients, Viagra test subjects got a "big surprise." Unfortunately, there is also research that Viagra increases clotting activity.[7] Elevated clotting agents increase heart attack risk. If you're at risk, Viagra isn't the safest choice.

Nitrates aren't any better. Doctors prescribe nitrate drugs for people with chest pain. They open vessels to allow blood to reach the heart easier. But they also damage the lining of your blood vessels.

Ironically, the drugs designed to improve blood flow may also damage it. And this zaps your strength and potency even more.

It's not just a bedroom issue. A lack of potency gives you the feeling that your whole body has gone limp. You lose your sense of power, your ability to do everyday activities – even getting out of bed can become a chore.

You can trigger the production of NO with a few simple

supplements. You'll get bigger blood flow, regardless of your current age or level of conditioning.

Use Nature's Viagra for Bigger, Better Blood Flow

The first step to more NO (and huge blood flow) is a simple amino acid called *l-arginine*. This building block is a precursor to nitric oxide. That means your body uses it to create NO.

Body builders have been using l-arginine for years. Taken before a workout, it gives them a "muscle pump" by dilating blood vessels and getting more blood and oxygen to their muscles.

L-arginine is an easy way to build new muscle, boost strength and stamina during your workout and speed recovery after your workout. Getting your body to make more NO ramps up your potency level. It's like a wave of "can do" energy that wakes you up across the board.

Your circulation will improve too. You'll notice a big difference – especially if you have trouble breathing. Many of my patients tell me they can take bigger, deeper breaths after taking l-arginine.

They tell me it feels like a power boost that affects their whole body. All at once they feel stronger, more alert and more alive.

There's a strong mental component to this experience too. All that extra blood and oxygen to your brain gives you the feeling of clarity and mental calm.

I've been using l-arginine for years. It's one of the most reliable, fast-acting tools for giving your manhood a boost fast. It's hard to underestimate the benefits (and pleasure) of getting more NO to your cells.

L-arginine is so essential, the guys who discovered the functions of nitric oxide were jointly awarded the 1998 Nobel Prize in Medicine.

They revealed NO's ability to send signals to your cells. Think of NO as a kind of "sex messenger," telling your blood vessels to expand. They also provided indisputable evidence that l-arginine is your body's chief source for creating nitric oxide.

To maintain healthy muscles, prevent heart disease, and stave off erectile dysfunction, you can take l-arginine in a capsule form. Take a 500 mg cap each day for prevention.

To boost your PACE performance, you'll get the most from l-arginine if you take it in powder form. To build lost muscle, improve sexual performance, or reduce chest pains, take up to 5 grams each day.

Because l-arginine is an amino acid, proteins compete with its absorption. For this reason, you shouldn't take it with meals. Instead, take it between meals on a relatively empty stomach. Simply take a teaspoon of powder and mix it with water.

Get Hard, New Muscle Without Lifting Weights

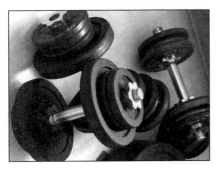

PACE is one of the most reliable ways to build new muscle. You don't need heavy weights or grueling gym routines. But there is a supplement that speeds the process. It's been an open secret in the bodybuilding world for years.

Just a few grams of this safe and reliable powder can add up to 10 pounds of new muscle – with almost no effort on your part.

Building up muscle is critical for virility and potency. Part of the "whole body erectile dysfunction" I spoke about earlier comes from your skeletal muscles becoming small, weak and powerless.

Skeletal muscles are the ones you can see, and the ones you exercise when you move. They attach to your bones via tendons and power up your whole body.

Strong skeletal muscles fill you with strength and potential. They give you the feeling of confidence and they ensure you stay mobile and independent. And they play a lead role in your metabolism.

Lose muscle, and fat takes its place… it's a tell-tale sign of old age.

Stop Muscle Loss – Even Reverse It – With *Creatine*

Professional athletes have been using creatine to naturally enhance their performance for years. Top athletes credit this supplement for allowing them to sprint faster, jump further, and lift heavier weights.

A baseball player I know told me creatine added 5 mph to his fastball, another athlete said it took a half second off his 100-meter sprint and a power lifter claimed it added 40 pounds to his bench press.

Vince Andrich, a nutrition adviser to athletes and author of *Sports Supplement Review,* was skeptical when he first heard about creatine. But that was before he tried it. After following a recommended regimen, he gained 10 pounds of new muscle in 2 weeks.

But did this added muscle actually make him stronger? In his words "*my strength went through the roof.*"[8]

Creatine Can Help You, Too

You may not throw a fastball, but you need strength in your arms to carry groceries, lift your grandkids and get stuff out of the trunk.

You may have no interest in running a 100-yard sprint, but having power in your legs is essential. It gets you out of bed in the morning, gets you through a round of golf, and keeps you out of a wheelchair.

"I was very skeptical before trying PACE… Everyone in the world wants you to believe that their system will help you lose weight and feel great. But instead of just making claims, Dr. Sears gave me a plan… and guess what, it worked!

After 5 months, I lost 33 lbs. of fat, and I've kept it off for 2 years now! I've never felt stronger and more alive – PACE actually works. I'll never go back to regular cardio – those days are over!"

Dave B., Denver, CO

Clinical Proof Creatine Boosts Athletic Performance

Your liver produces creatine, but 98% of it is stored in your skeletal muscle. Creatine serves as an instant source of energy for muscle contraction. The ability to quickly contract your muscles is critical for success when performing a short-duration exercise like sprinting or weightlifting.[9]

Another important function of creatine is its ability to block or buffer hydrogen ions. Hydrogen ions are a sprinter's or power lifter's enemy. Hydrogen ions cause the pH of muscles cells to become more acidic. Acidic pH causes muscles to fatigue.

When you perform several short sessions of intense anaerobic exercise like sprinting or lifting barbells, a rapid depletion of your creatine starts within seconds, along with an increase in hydrogen ions.

This is why you feel the burn of exhaustion in your muscles when pushing them to complete a set of exercises like bicep curls or pushups.

Studies on lab rats revealed those rats who received creatine supplementation ran faster and longer than rats without supplementation. A Nottingham, England study at Queen's Medical Center revealed that oral supplementation of creatine increased muscle creatine uptake by 50%.[10]

A study from Texas Southwestern Medical Center and The Cooper Clinic confirmed creatine's performance ability. All participants were experienced weight trainers. They took 20 grams of creatine for 28 days. The researchers then measured their single-rep maximum bench press.

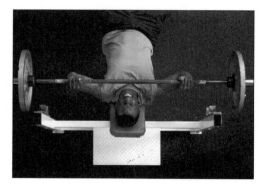

On average, they lifted 18 pounds more than the control group in only 28 days of training.[11]

How to Maximize the Benefits of Creatine in Your PACE Workout

Although you get some creatine from red meat, it's not enough to create a "creatine loading effect." You would have to eat 9 pounds of meat a day to get 20 grams of creatine.

You need a creatine supplement if you want to maximize the strength benefits. The following chart will assist you in determining your personal loading dose and maintenance dose:

Your Creatine Loading and Maintenance Doses		
Lean Body Mass in lbs.	**Loading Dose in Grams**	**Maintenance in Grams**
100	10	5
120	10	5
140	12.5	5
160	15	7.5
180	17.5	7.5
200	20	10

Modified by Dr. Sears from: The Colgan Institute, San Diego.

Notice the doses are in grams not milligrams so capsules are ineffective. Buy creatine as 100% pure powder, mix it with water and drink immediately. One teaspoon is 5 grams and one tablespoon is 15 grams.

Don't fall for the marketing publicity. Pure creatine is all you need. You don't need a carbohydrate load like some sellers of creatine drinks claim and the gels are no better than the inexpensive powder. The best time to take it is 30 to 60 minutes before PACE but you will still benefit from other dosing times.

I recommend taking a loading dose for 10 days. Then continue with the maintenance dose for 3 months. After a 3-month cycle, you have two options. You can stop and use exercise to maintain your gains in performance and lean muscle. Or you can switch back to the loading dose for 10 days again and repeat the cycle.

Remember, you need PACE to realize the benefits of creatine. It won't work its magic by sitting on the couch.

There are two potential side effects of creatine you should be aware of, but neither is serious and they are both reversible.

Some researchers have found a slightly increased rate of muscle cramping with creatine. Others disagree. If you get muscle cramps, stop the creatine for a week and then begin again at half the dose. Massage the muscle that cramped to stimulate circulation before each exercise session.

Other athletes, especially sprinters have reported nausea during exercise after taking creatine. If you should get this, try eating a couple of slices of pineapple or papaya after taking your creatine.

Another concern you should be aware of when supplementing with creatine is to go light on the caffeine. Caffeine and creatine don't mix well. Some studies suggest that caffeine (a common performance enhancer among athletes) may diminish the effectiveness of creatine if taken at the same time.

Overall, it is very well tested, all natural, and has an exceptional safety record. If you use it intelligently, creatine can enhance your athletic performance, strength and virility, and help to increase your lean body mass.

Endnotes

1 Rasmussen BB, Tipton KD, Miller SL, Wolf SE, Wolfe RR.. An oral essential amino acid-carbohydrate supplement enhances muscle protein anabolism after resistance exercise. *J Appl Physiol*. 2000;88(2): 386 - 392.

2 Horrocks L, Yeo YK. Health benefits of docosahexaenoic acid. *Pharmacol Res*. 1999;40(3): 211-225.

3 Hope BK, Baker R, Edel ED, et al. An overview of the salmonella enteritidis risk assessment for shell, egg, and egg products. *Risk Anal* 2002;22(2): 203-218.

4 Frank B. *Forever Young*: 100 Age-Erasing Techniques. New York, NY: Harper Collins, 2003:30-31.

5 Boyle M. *Personal Nutrition*. 4th ed, Belmont, CA: Wadsworth/Thomson Learning.

6 Ibid

7 Li Z, Xi X, Gu M, et al. A stimulatory role for cGMP-dependent protein kinase in platelet activation. *Cell* 2003;112(1):77-86.

8 Andrich, V. *Sports Supplement Review*. 3rd issue, Mile High Publishing:48.

9 Weider Research Group. Creatine: The Science Behind bodybuilding's most popular supplement. *Muscle & Fitness*. 1998: 146-148.

10 Colgan, M. Dr. Colgan's Best Body Supplements: Creatine. *All Natural Muscular Development*. 1998;35(3):90-94.

11 Ibid.

CHAPTER TWELVE

PACE for Life

In an ideal world you wouldn't need PACE. In fact, you wouldn't need any kind of exercise at all.

As you've discovered, the bodies of our ancestors were seamlessly connected to their environment. They instinctively followed life's demands and natural cycles. And their bodies responded in kind.

PACE rekindles those instincts by putting you back in touch with the cycles of health and fitness. By now you're already familiar with the most important patterns and natural cycles for staying fit and lean:

- Exertion and recovery
- Progressive changes
- Adaptive responses
- Breaking plateaus
- Functional strength through daily life

In this chapter, I'll take you deeper into PACE by fine tuning your practice and adding elements that bring it all together. You'll discover the subtleties of breathing, the nature of cycles, and the practicalities of goal setting.

I discovered some of these subtle yet powerful secrets after working with PACE for years. Let me start by introducing you to one of the great pioneers in the largely ignored science of health enhancing cycles. This pioneering cardiologist and researcher confirmed PACE principles in a way that's both unique and startling.

Olympic Committee Chairman
Makes Gold Medal Discovery

Dr. Irving Dardik was the first Chairman of the U.S. Olympic Committee's Sports Medicine Council. His revelation illustrates the core principles of PACE. And clearly details its power to reverse chronic diseases as diverse as Parkinson's, diabetes, multiple sclerosis and arthritis.

The story begins with Dr. Dardik's friend Jack Kelly. Jack was the brother of actress Grace Kelly. He was also an Olympic oarsman and, at the time, the president of the U.S. Olympic Committee. One morning he went out for his usual run and, shortly after, dropped dead of sudden heart failure.

Dr. Dardik knew that heart attacks often occur **after** running or jogging – not during the workout. He added, *"People have been running for thousands of years, and they didn't die like that. It must be something in the way people run now that causes heart failure after exertion."* [1]

He also observed long-distance runners were prone to infections and chronic diseases, especially heart disease. He compared their exercise practices to the habits of native people and animals.

He said animals and natives in the wild run in short bursts. Then, they take time for recovery. And, they repeat this cycle of exertion and recovery.

"Cheetahs, the fastest creatures on Earth, run in short bursts... And I found that all animals do that: a burst of exertion, then rest; a burst of exertion, then rest. You see this in whales when they dive, sharks when they hunt, birds in flight.

Everywhere I looked, no matter what kind of animal was involved, it was the same pattern: a burst of exertion, followed by rest, and so on. You see it in young children, as well, when they are playing. They run. They stop. They run. They stop. This mode of exertion, which seems to be nature's way, these kids do it naturally – until we start training them in athletics, that is."

He concluded long-distance runners die of heart attacks because they don't train their hearts to recover. This is the same conclusion I made in my own book, **The Doctor's Heart Cure**.[2]

"Since implementing PACE, I have cut my workout from 45-60 minutes on the cross trainer down to 22 minutes and burn more fat calories. I burn 61 fat calories in 22 minutes and have reduced my 'belly fat' substantially. I am 52-years-old and feel as though I am back in my late 20s."

Brett K., Ft. McMurray, Alberta, Canada

Reconnecting With Nature's Rhythms and Cycles: Your *Heart Wave*

These observations led Dr. Dardik to his fascinating concept of viewing heart exertion and recovery as a wave – the "Heart Wave." When you begin exercise, your heart rate begins to climb. When you stop, it begins to come back down. Think about that. If you plot these changing rates going up, then down, through time, it does indeed form a wave.

Inside that wave of exertion, you have smaller waves from each heartbeat – itself an alternating wave of exertion (systole) and recovery (diastole). Dardik was the first to see these as "waves within waves." The picture below will help you visualize the concept.

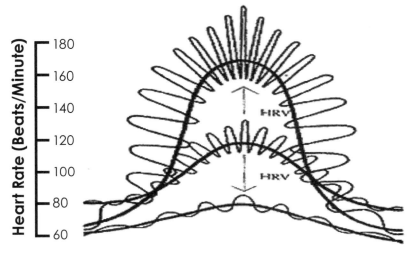

The central wave represents your heart rate increasing with exertion and dropping with recovery. The smaller waves represent each heartbeat as it contracts and releases with its own wave of exertion and recovery.

Adapted from Irving J. Dardik. "The Origin of Disease and Health: Heart Waves." Cycles, Vol. 46, No. 3, 1996

Reverse Disease With Stronger Heart Waves

If you mimic the natural rhythms of your heart by exercising in intervals of exertion and recovery, you gradually increase your *heart rate variability*, or HRV. Simply stated, the greater your HRV, the better your overall health. The more limited your HRV, the greater your risk of chronic disease.

During his research, the non-athletic people Dr. Dardik studied significantly increased their heart rate variability. They also gained:

- greater lung volume
- lower blood pressure
- improved immune function
- lower stress and anxiety
- greater sense of energy and well-being

All of these changes happened in just 8 weeks. To quote Dardik, *"Cyclic exercise really worked in reversing disease."* [3]

Think of HRV as your ability to experience a wide range of heart rates. Imagine going from a resting rate of 80 bpm all the way up to 190 bpm in a matter of a few minutes. Then back to resting just as quickly.

Most of us don't have that degree of variability. Our heartbeat mostly stays inside a narrow band: We get out of bed, we go to work, we sit at a desk, we come home, we sit on a couch. That kind of activity does not challenge the heart or give it room for changing speeds.

Aerobics and cardio are guilty of the same non-variation. When we exercise aerobically, our heart rate also stays within a narrow band, just at a different speed than resting.

Mainstream medicine accepts the fact that HRV is a risk factor for both infectious and chronic diseases. They don't know why, but clinical studies confirm it.

Decades of research has shown that increased HRV is associated with longevity and non-disease states. Likewise, decreased HRV is associated with disease and a high risk of death from all causes.

Think about this for a moment. When your heart has the capacity to jump into high gear whenever it needs to… and then recover at a moment's notice, you are in excellent health. Your heart can pump blood and oxygen quickly and without effort. You have power on demand and the ability to adapt and turn on a dime.

> *"I love what you have taught me with PACE. After just a few weeks, I built up my lung capacity again, and my strength."*
>
> Jane M., El Sobrante, CA

When your heart doesn't have the capacity to beat faster with any amount of certainty or reliability, you're in trouble. That's the power of HRV.

Here's an excerpt from one of Dr. Dardik's journal articles.[4] In it he describes how modern exercise trains us to lower our HRV, which actually boosts our risk of disease.

> *"A decrease in Heart Wave range is equivalent to a pianist trying to play a piano concerto using only one octave of a piano's full range. Just as a decrease in the Heart Wave range (decreased HRV) leads to decreased longevity and chronic disease, expanding the Heart Wave range (increased HRV) leads to increased longevity and health.*
>
> *In this regard, the implications for fitness training are significant. When we speak of fitness, we infer a positive relationship between fitness and health; fitness should cause good health. However, this is not always the case. In fact, there are reports that suggest an association between continuous, long duration exercise with infectious diseases including polio, echoviral meningitis, respiratory and gastrointestinal infections as well as with cancer, cardio-vascular disease, and multiple sclerosis.[5][6][7][8][9]*
>
> *This association between fitness training and chronic disorders can now be explained by recognizing that prolonged continuous*

*training in a narrow target heart rate zone, through aerobic exercise or any other form of linear stress, actually will train HRV to decrease. The same would apply to any behavior done in a continuous fashion. By teaching HRV to become more linear, more even – in other words, flattening the Heart Waves – **the individual is actually training to become more susceptible to chronic disease and all cause mortality**.* (Emphasis added.)

Instead of linear aerobic fitness, which is designed to push the limits of oxygen consumption (VO$_2$max) but ignores oxygen recovery, we should be training the Heart Wave range to expand. In fact, physical fitness (like energy) generally is described as 'the ability to work.' What this definitely does not take into account is 'the ability not to work' – i.e., recovery."

In other words, when you practice long-duration exercise and ignore recovery you make your body weaker, more prone to disease and more likely to die young.

There's no doubt: PACE increases your heart rate variability or HRV. In just minutes a day you can program your body for longevity and disease prevention.

Dr. Dardik's research is remarkable. However, he did miss one point when it comes to fitness and training. And that's *progressivity*.

Keeping your HRV high means changing up your routine and adding new elements that progressively increase the challenge. In this way, PACE is a complete program. It's self-contained and has all the elements you need for a lifetime of strength and vigor.

Explore Nature's Other Life Cycle: Breathing

Martial artists, yoga masters and high-level athletes from

around the world have a secret weapon. It's what Bruce Lee called "Breath Power," the ability to control your breathing patterns to improve strength, stamina and sense of well being.

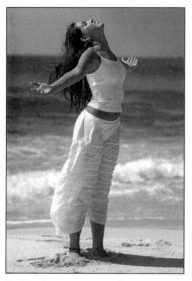

When you're practicing PACE, awareness and control of your breath will take you to a deeper and more advanced level of achievement.

Besides delivering oxygen to your muscles during exertion, breathing is also the foundation for emotional intensity, physical equilibrium, and a sense of internal power.

Martial artists and high performance athletes of all kinds know that proper breathing techniques help them get in the zone, perform better and recover much more quickly.

On top of that, improving your breathing literally helps improve your ability to develop higher and higher levels of functional fitness.

In addition to their role in bringing the air in and out of our lungs, the breathing muscles (principally the diaphragm, the muscles of the rib cage and the abdominal muscles) play a vital role in stabilizing and rotating the upper body.

So in essence, the quality of your breathing directly affects your core strength and lays the foundation for optimal athletic performance.

What Are the Benefits of Proper Breathing During PACE?

Hundreds of studies have proven that proper breathing techniques before, during and after exercise deliver:

- increased stamina
- increased endurance
- better performance
- quicker recovery
- enhanced oxygen absorption
- increased muscle development

Proper breathing provides your body with oxygen for the correct and efficient functioning of every cell. Without sufficient oxygen, your muscles cannot perform at their peak, leaving you weak and listless part way through your workout.

Additionally, improper breathing inhibits your cells from metabolizing your food properly. That means all those nutrients and vitamins you need to build, tone and repair your muscles will be lost.

Proper breathing, on the other hand, allows your body to metabolize food efficiently and to rid itself of all the noxious, gaseous by-products of metabolism, especially carbon dioxide.

Proper breathing soothes the nervous system; calms, steadies, and clears the mind; improves concentration; focuses attention; and increases the ability to deal with complex situations without suffering from stress. Plus, it tones and trains your diaphragm, rib and abdominal muscles to improve core strength and stability.

Use These 4 Basic Breathing Techniques Today

Depending on whom you talk with, there are hundreds of different breathing techniques to choose from. But for the sake of simplicity, we'll discuss four main breathing methods that have proven to help athletes improve stamina and strength.

Focused Breathing — Most experts agree that for optimal health, your breathing should be full and rhythmic, using your diaphragm and ribs to fill and empty the lungs.

Your diaphragm is a large muscle that rests horizontally across the base of your rib cage. (Imagine an inflated parachute attached all around your lower rib cage.) The diaphragm is connected in the front, along the sides of your lower ribs, and along the back.

This type of deep abdominal breathing promotes a full exchange of air, keeping the oxygen/carbon dioxide ratio in your body balanced. Focused breathing utilizes this deep natural breathing pattern to develop rhythm and muscle focus while exercising.

Focused breathing should be deep and natural, with no impediments. The trick is to keep your mind focused on your breathing and on the muscles you are training.

For example, when doing squats or deep knee bends, you would inhale slowly as you descend then exhale as you rise to a standing position. You'll want to be sure to breathe in through your nose to strengthen your diaphragm and exhale through your mouth to alleviate pressure.

For pushups, simply inhale as you descend, exhale as you push your body up, using the same in through the nose out through the mouth technique described above.

Focused breathing is essential for proper development of your abdominals as well. Many people "forget" to breathe when doing sit-ups or abdominal crunches and lose much of the benefit of training. For maximum effect, inhale at your resting position and exhale as you contract your abdominal muscles.

To increase your benefits, sharpen your mental focus. For maximum muscle gain, focus your mind on the muscles you're training. See them contracting and relaxing as you rhythmically breathe in and out. The connection between your mind and body while performing this breathing technique produces improved performance and overall muscle gain.

Using this focused breathing technique enhances your ability to perform each movement and will increase your fitness results over time.

> *"I am a 58-year-old male with type-2 diabetes and cardiovascular disease (CVD). I began PACE in January 2009 and the results have been no less than incredible. My weight has dropped 11 lbs., body fat dropped from 30% to 22%, and lost 3 inches off waist. Thanks to Dr. Sears' programs and advice, I believe I am on the right track to good health for the foreseeable future."*
>
> Kiel B., Land O Lakes, FL

Bellows Breath — The Bellows Breath is an adaptation of an ancient yoga breathing technique revered for its ability to increase energy and a sense of well being. Incorporate the Bellows Breath technique before or after your PACE workout to improve cardiovascular function and to recover more quickly.

Begin by sitting in a comfortable position. Take a few deep breaths through your nose filling the lungs from bottom to the top

– like a glass of water (expanding your abdomen and then filling the top of the lungs). Exhale through the nostrils doing the exact opposite. Expel the air from top to bottom, forcing the last of the air out with your abdomen pressing in.

After 2 to 3 warm up breaths, try blowing little puffs of air through your nostrils as you exhale. This should feel like a series of short, staccato exhalations, flexing your abdominal muscles inward with each short exhale. Be sure not to go too fast. After 15 to 20 repetitions, let your breathing return to normal.

The Bellows Breath technique will improve your stamina, overall concentration and sense of well being. It will "clear your head" and might even improve your cognitive abilities as well!

Lung Expansion — In this exercise, you will use deep diaphragmatic breathing to increase your lung capacity and to super oxygenate your muscles before and after a PACE workout.

When you inhale, the diaphragm muscle pulls downward, so that the ribs flare out slightly, while the bottom of your lungs pull downward to bring in air. With deep diaphragmatic breathing, the space just below the breastbone, at the upper abdomen pushes in slightly to exhale more completely.

Inhale and exhale deeply pulling your shoulders back as you do. This will open up your lung cavity and allow your lungs to expand. Do 3 to 5 lung expansion breaths before and after each exercise to oxygenate your muscles and to shorten your recovery time.

Power Breathing — Use this technique to improve your actual strength while performing bodyweight calisthenics.

Unlike the previous forms of diaphragmatic breathing we've

discussed, which require you to exhale completely, power breathing does not.

Power breathing is a method to increase the pressure in your abdomen to stimulate additional strength at the moment of exertion. If you've ever watched Olympic weight lifting or a martial arts competition, you've seen power breathing at work.

Here's how it works. Right before you perform a calisthenic exercise, inhale deeply through your nose. Be sure to breathe down into your abdomen and not just your chest. You'll know you're doing it right when you see your abdomen expand slightly as you inhale.

Next, hold your breath as you begin the exercise. Then as you begin to exert force, increase your abdominal pressure slightly. You'll probably feel the need to grunt, that's okay. Keep up the abdominal pressure through the full range of motion, then release.

> **Special Note:** Consult your doctor before performing this breathing technique if you have high blood pressure, heart problems, hernias or other health concerns.

There you have it. A quick primer on how to improve your breathing that will help you increase your natural stamina, strength and overall lungpower. Now let's have a look at setting goals and turning knowledge into action.

Bringing It All Together
Good Planning Is the Key to Success

Deep down, I know I'd be lazy if I allowed myself to be that way. My natural inclination is to procrastinate. But because I recognize this shortcoming, I've developed a system that makes health improving habits *automatic*.

If you will get started now and follow this specific plan of action… it will ensure that you don't put off your most important step – the actual doing.

Every important accomplishment I have ever made started with planning. Every night, I take five minutes and plan my exercises and meals for the next day. I don't always stick to it, but without a plan, I tend to miss workouts and eat whatever is available. I don't bother with detail and I don't feel guilty if it changes. I think of it as a self-coaching tool.

Let's say tomorrow is Monday… I know I will be very busy with patients at the clinic and have several meetings afterwards. So I plan a brief PACE workout before going to the office, and strength training at lunch. Otherwise, I know I'll never get it done.

For breakfast, I'll have eggs and some left-over salmon from tonight's dinner. For lunch, I'll order a seafood salad to-go from the restaurant near the gym. I take some steaks out of the freezer to thaw for dinner.

Early to Bed, Early to Rise

Ben Franklin was right. Getting up early is profoundly health enhancing. I incorporate this in my routine.

6:00 AM: My alarm sounds. I put some motivation near the alarm the night before. Since I am in a leaning down cycle, I have my body composition log and my running equipment as the first thing I see. This makes it impossible to forget my goal and my motivation. I have a cup of coffee while I read my email. It's now 6:45 AM and the sun is rising as I walk out the door.

I follow my PACE program for cardio. As you already know, the principle is to build larger lung and heart capacity. To accomplish this, I provide my heart and lungs with short challenges just above my capacity to sustain.

When I stop to catch my breath, I know I've provided that little excess challenge. By doing this a little bit every day, I gradually build reserve capacity.

Today I've decided to bicycle. I start with a 2-minute warm up at a gentle pace. I then accelerate to a moderate 5 out of 10 rating for 1 minute. I then drop back down to a 3 rating for 1 minute of recovery. I repeat this cycle 3 more times advancing to 6, 7, and 8 ratings for about a minute followed by a minute of recovery while I pedal at a 3 or 4 rating and breathe deeply.

Feels good today! For my last exertion period, I'm going to give it everything I have. I pedal as hard as I can for 30 seconds. I feel an intense burn in the front of my thighs as I move into my supra-aerobic zone. I know my body will get the message to improve my oxygen delivering capacity.

Warm-Up	Set 1		Set 2	
	Exertion	Recovery	Exertion	Recovery
2 min	1 min	1 min	1 min	1 min

Set 3		Set 4		Set 5	
Exertion	Recovery	Exertion	Recovery	Exertion	Recovery
45 sec	1 min	45 sec	1 min	30 sec	1 min

I think about how important quads are to physical capacity as I am panting during recovery.

Your quadriceps muscle is the largest in your body. It requires the most fuel. I pedal easily back to my house. Total time: 12 minutes.

Load Up on Protein for Breakfast

Breakfast is a 3-egg omelet, salmon and water. I put 10 grams of glutamine in my water. It prevents muscle breakdown and boosts growth hormone. I take 1000-mg of Vitamin C and a combinational multi-vitamin, multi-mineral, multi-antioxidant supplement with my breakfast.

I have 2 basic rules to guide my eating. One, I don't eat food I don't like. I don't care who says it's good for me. Two, I try to eat only food that occurs naturally. Eating food that occurs naturally can be a challenge. Most modern food is man-made or adulterated in one way or another.

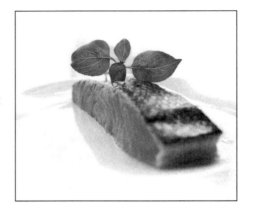

After breakfast, I spend 20 minutes on calisthenics. First, I do one of my favorites, Hindu squats. To build strength in the legs and back – and boost your lung volume – this exercise can't be beat. Today, I'll just do 75 – although on some days, I'll push myself and do 500.

I follow this with crunches, push-ups and instep touches. In just a few minutes, I've worked my entire body. As part of a regular rou-

tine, this is the best way to build muscle. It also develops the kind of functional strength that keeps you fit and mobile past 100.

It's time to shower, and get to the office...

Calisthenics Training Log		
Muscles Worked	**Exercise**	**Reps**
Legs, Gluteus	Hindu Squats	25 – 25 – 25
Abs, Lower Back	Crunches/Sit Ups	15 – 15 – 15
Upper Body	Push Ups	10 – 10
Full Body	Instep Touches	10 – 10

Reliable Energy for the Afternoon

I stop by a local restaurant and place an order for a seafood salad to-go. I ask them to add an extra portion of grilled dolphin to the salad. Since I'm working the big muscles of the legs today, I want extra protein after my workout.

I meet with my research assistant while I eat mixed seafood and spinach, then it's time to see patients.

After 2 hours of patients, I retreat to my office for a few minutes. I listen to music, drink a fruit smoothie and snack on some cheese. I finish with my patients, have a brief meeting with a perspective new employee for the Wellness Research Foundation and another with my office manager and it's off to baseball practice.

I take the kids through some calisthenics. Exercising with 8-year-olds has turned out to be great fun and I get to spend more time with my son. One hour to practice basic throwing, catching and hitting and it's home for dinner.

The Most Complete Nutrition Source

Despite the constant droning over the dangers of red meat, I eat it just about every day. In our natural environment, approximately 85% of our total calories came from red meat. Red meat is the highest quality nutrition – bar none.

In our modern world though, if you eat any animal you have to concern yourself with the environment of that animal. It makes all the difference in the world.

Keeping animals inactive and feeding them grains does the same thing to them that it does to us. It makes them obese with all the wrong kind of fat.

I much prefer **grass-fed** beef or wild game. It's full of heart-healthy nutrients with none of the hormones and antibiotics that can threaten your health. I have found wild game from a local hunting group. You can find out more about grass-fed beef at my website: www.alsearsmd.com.

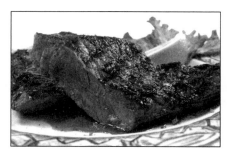

Today it's T-bones on the grill. I also grill up some onions and bell peppers. In Florida, we have tomatoes ripe now. I pick one yellow tomato and two red beefsteak tomatoes from my back yard. I wash and slice them and dinner is ready. I enjoy my steak and vegetables on the back patio with my family as the sun goes down.

I take another 1000 mg of vitamin C and 400 IU mixed tocopherols with dinner. I also take 100 mg of the ubiquinol form of Coenzyme Q10.

Hungry for Dessert? Eat Naturally Sweet

I have a bowl of ice cream with a sliced peach, hand-whipped cream and walnuts. I don't worry about fat but I do try to eat low glycemic fruit. Peaches have a glycemic index lower than whole wheat bread. I also buy ice cream without added sugar. You can get it from most grocery stores.

	Meal Log	Supplements
Breakfast	Cup of Coffee, 3 egg omelet, salmon, water	Glutamine 10 gm Vit C 1000 mg Multivitamin
Lunch	Seafood salad with extra grilled dolphin and spinach	
Afternoon Snack	Fruit Smoothie, cheese	
Dinner	Grilled grass-fed steak, onions, bell peppers, tomatoes	Vit C 1000 mg Tocopherols 400 IU Co Q10 100 mg
Evening Snack	Bowl of ice cream with a sliced peach and walnuts	

Quiet Reflection... Exercise for the Soul

Freud said we need three things to be happy: relationships, occupation and recreation. In other words, we need to love, work, and play. Under the stress of our modern lifestyle, we tend to focus nearly all of our energy for change on our careers. When that happens, we often neglect relationships and recreation.

I take a contemplative walk around my neighborhood. This is not real physical exercise and most people get plenty of walking during their daily routine but it does allow me to relax. Afterwards, I may watch some TV or read.

I think it is a mistake to treat your health and fitness goals as you do your occupation. I do not consider a health improving lifestyle to be work. It's part of my recreation. Plan it in the same spirit you would plan a mini-vacation. I also try to involve family and friends whenever possible.

11:00 PM: Time to hit the sack. I think for a few minutes about what I'd like to accomplish tomorrow. What I would like to eat and how I feel about exercise. I jot it down in my log. I clear my mind and reflect for a few minutes. Now, I get to bed early.

Chart Your Daily Action Plan

- Make your plan for eating and exercise the day before.
- Focus your plan on exercise you enjoy and eat only the natural foods you like.
- Start the day right with brief cardio exercise before breakfast.
- Eat a high protein breakfast.
- Train for strength either before lunch or before dinner.
- Make a portion of your physical activity recreation every day.
- Plan dinner around high quality protein (steak, roast, fish, chicken).
- Involve your family and your friends.
- Reflect on today's progress and plan for tomorrow's.

I credit my good health to my daily habits. No one will ever convince me otherwise. But having said that, I don't beat myself up if I slip. I am not perfect and I suspect you aren't either. You won't succeed everyday and you shouldn't expect to.

Remember, excellent health is more of a journey than a destination. So be sure to enjoy the trip…

Endnotes

1 Lewin R. Tuning Biorhythms through Cyclic Exercise. *Holistic Primary Care*. 2006:7(1):1

2 Sears Al. *The Doctor's Heart Cure*. St. Paul, MN:Dragon Door Publications;2004.

3 Lewin R. *Making Waves: Irving Dardik and his Superwave Principle*. Rodale Books;2005

4 Dardik IJ. The Origin of Disease and Health: Heart Waves – the Single Solution to Heart Rate Variability and Ischemic Preconditioning; *Cycles*, Vol. 46, No. 3, 1996.

5 Sharp C, Parry-Billings M. Can exercise damage your health? Athletes who train hard seem to unusually prone to illness. But the complexities of the immune system make it difficult to understand why. *New Scientist*, pp. 33-37, August 15, 1992.

6 Burfoot A. How Much Should You Run? *Runner's World*, pp. 66-67, September 1995.

7 Martin S. Heart sick: why are the hearts of top riders failing – and what does it mean for you? *Bicycling*, pp. 58-61, August 1995.

8 Kanter E. Sharing Gold Medals, and Multiple Sclerosis. *The New York Times*, p. 11, June 25, 1995.

9 National Center for Health Statistics. Physical activity and health: a report of the Surgeon General; July 11, 1996.

PACE Workbook

Guarantee Your Success:
Keep a Record of Everything You Do

As a life-long "health nut," athlete, sports trainer, consultant, personal fitness trainer and integrative doctor, I've worked with thousands of people. I have found no better predictor of who will be successful at reaching their goals than whether or not they are willing to keep a log. If you want progress, write down what you do.

I have included workbook pages from my own log on a special website. I also use it for planning. I pencil it in and then write over it in pen when I actually do it.

Okay, enough talk. Let's get down to it.

Here's a link where you'll find workbook pages you can download and use with PACE:

www.pacerevolution.com/workbook

Visit this website and get started today. Everything you need to set your PACE goals and track your progress is right there. Don't wait.

Take the Guesswork Out of PACE

Nothing helps you get results faster than seeing PACE demonstrated on video. So I asked my PACE trainers to show you exactly what to do.

Go to the exclusive website below and you'll see and hear all the routines in Chapter 9 explained in detail. We'll demonstrate all the calisthenics and body weight exercises. It's all right here:

www.pacerevolution.com/video

No more guesswork. You have all the tools you need to start doing PACE right now.

APPENDIX B

Common PACE
Questions Answered

Endurance Plus PACE

Q: *"Dr. Sears, I run marathons. Can I still do PACE? And can I use PACE to help me train for endurance events?"*

A: Many people think that PACE means that they have to give up all endurance training. This is understandable since I often point out the weaknesses in endurance training. But actually PACE and marathons are not mutually exclusive.

In fact, PACE will help you tolerate the endurance training you need for a marathon while giving up less of your heart strength and lungpower. I've also seen the combination of PACE and endurance training work well in athletes from tennis players to wrestlers who need a combination of both endurance and explosive strength.

The key is using PACE effectively to build up your cardiopulmonary capacity. Using a PACE routine will boost your lung volume and achieve a higher cardiac output – which is precisely what marathon runners who train only for endurance are missing.

If you train ONLY for endurance, you'll lose lung volume and your heart will slowly shrink, causing your maximal achievable heart and lung output to drop. This will weaken your performance whenever you need bursts of high energy activity or strength. What's worse, is it will threaten your health over the long term by accelerating losses of aging and making you more prone to heart attack and stroke.

By supplementing your endurance training with a PACE routine, you'll actually improve a broader range of athletic capabilities. At the same time, you'll build and retain the heart and lung strength of youth.

Lance Armstrong is a most excellent example. He is principally an endurance athlete yet he uses high-intensity sprints as part of his regular workout routine. And he puts a great deal of emphasis on building lung volume and VO_2max, (the highest rate of oxygen consumption attainable during maximal or exhaustive exercise...) – each of which are critical to both your athletic performance and your long-term health.

Here's how to make PACE work with your endurance training:

- First you will have to (for a time) limit your endurance training. If you are not willing to at least temporarily limit the frequency of endurance training – say running more than a mile continuously – you are not likely to make good progress at building your heart and lung capacity or strength.

- Next, measure your heart's recovery time. Start by logging your resting heart rate. Record your heart rate at the end of your PACE exertion set and make note of how long it takes you to get back to a rate within 10 beats of your resting heart rate.

- Practice a short PACE routine of only 12 minutes, 3 times a week, for an 8-week block. During this time, focus on increasing your maximal exertion. Slowly and gradually work up to higher and higher speeds for brief exertion sets of no more than 1 minute. Give yourself enough time between sets so that you get to within 10 beats of your resting heart rate.

- Monitor your recovery heart rate throughout the 8 week block. You should notice your recovery time getting shorter and shorter over this 2-month period even though you are working at a higher level of exertion.
- Practice your endurance routine only once every 2 weeks.

You may have some resistance to cutting back on your endurance training. But if you can have a little faith, your payoff will be huge. When you return to your usual training after an 8-week PACE training session, you'll notice a huge difference in your performance capacity.

Your lung volume and VO_2max will be considerably higher. Your heart's pumping power and output will soar. And this added capacity will make you more competitive.

As an added bonus, you'll probably drop body fat, and you are very likely to get a significant boost in your lean body mass.

How to Accelerate Your Fat Loss

Q: *"I'm interested in what Dr. Sears talked about for increasing the fat burning of the program."*

A: Here's how you can accelerate your fat loss... If you follow it for 2 to 3 weeks, you'll see dramatic changes.

Start by eliminating carbs and pumping up protein.

Here's how to make it work:

In the morning, start with a protein shake and throw in some raw eggs. You can use milk, juice or water – whichever you prefer. Mix in 2 scoops of whey protein isolate. That should give you at least 50 mg of protein. Add 2 raw eggs. Stir and drink up.

That extra protein tells your body that "the hunting is good," and signals your body to start burning off fat. The raw eggs, aside from proving the perfect ratio of amino acids, also give you the right kind of fat – triggering even more fat loss.

You can also cook some eggs and have them with grass fed steak or bacon. But try and keep carbs out of your breakfast in the morning.

In the afternoon, stay with lean protein. For this program, raw foods are best but not mandatory. If you like sashimi or sushi, that makes a great lunch.

If raw is not your thing, try cooked fish and/or meat. But no bread or potatoes. Your carbs should come from vegetables. I find soups very good for lunch as long as they have no additives, sweeteners or high carb ingredients.

Raw foods may sound extreme, but your body can easily digest them. What's more, raw foods are packed with nutrients that are untouched and undamaged by the cooking process.

By giving your digestive system a break, you'll have a chance to get rid of accumulated waste in your colon. This also gets rid of extra bulk around your middle. Between meals, try a colon cleanser to help you with this.

In the evening, have another shake – the same one you prepared in the morning. Afterward, have a salad of mixed veggies. But avoid commercial, store-bought salad dressings. Stick to olive oil and balsamic vinegar or better yet – sacha inchi oil.

This may be a tough plan for you to follow, but it's not intended for more than a few weeks at a time. But if you can stick with it – and do your PACE program at the same time – you'll see incredible gains. Fat will start falling off your body.

You'll be amazed at how good you feel after just 14 days.

How Long Do You Maintain Maximum Exertion?

Q: *"Dr. Sears, how long do I maintain maximum exertion? I know I need to pant and create an oxygen deficit but I'm not clear on how long I maintain the highest-level exertion... Also: How low do I need to let my heart rate drop before doing my next exertion period? Does it need to drop by a certain number of beats, a percentage of how high it got, or just above my resting rate?"*

A: Your maximum exertion triggers many of the changes you want from your PACE program, including boosting your maximum metabolic rate. How long you maintain it during your exertion period is less important than achieving your highest rate because that's what will boost your performance capacity for next time.

You probably can only exert yourself at a maximum rate for short bursts of 20 to 30 seconds. This is a critical point, as some people don't push themselves to reach their maximum output during their PACE routine. It requires effort and on some days, you may not feel up to it. But keep in mind that PACE only requires maximum output for short periods.

How do you know if you're at your highest level of exertion?

Physically, your legs will burn, your heart will race and you'll feel as if you can't run another step. And when you stop, you'll feel winded and break into a pant.

If you're out of shape, your highest level of exertion may only last a few seconds. If this is the case, that's fine. As your lungs expand and your heart's pumping capacity increases, you'll be able to boost your maximum output soon enough.

It is the gradual progression of your highest level of exertion that is so effective for building a stronger heart and a bigger set of lungs. It also modifies your metabolic rate, helping you to burn calories as energy instead of storing them as fat.

Today, our most popular forms of exercise focus on constant exertion without rest. You repeat this enough and your body interprets this as chronic stress from a poor or unstable environment. This weakens your heart and shrinks your lung capacity. That in itself is a formula for heart attack and stroke.

Training your body to recover after exertion is essential for good health. It's a trait we've lost over time. But it's one of the capacities of a heart and lungs in top condition. Your ancient ancestors would have had this ability. Their daily activities demanded that they exert themselves in short bursts followed by rest. Hunting and fighting are good examples of how brief but intense their most important physical exertions would have been.

How Often Should You Do PACE?

Q: *"How many times a week do you suggest to do the program? For how long? And how often do I change the routine? Also, I use a rebounder. How can I apply your system with my equipment? I live in Canada and can't go out during the winter."*

A: I applaud your efforts to stay fit. Not only will PACE help you get the results you're looking for, you'll be able to do it in a fraction of the time you spent on longer routines.

Start by doing PACE at least 3 times a week. Put the emphasis on challenging your heart rate and finding your limits. Follow the workout times, but don't get stuck on them. They are guidelines, not hard and fast rules. Allow plenty of time for recovery. If you need more than the book suggests, then take time out and do it.

Increase the intensity each week. Push yourself to reach a little further each time you do the routine. If you feel like you need more, do it 4 or 5 times a week. But the core focus needs to be pushing for maximum exertion.

When you're done, you should feel like you've really done something. Your legs should ache and your shirt should be drenched in sweat. If you're not winded or if you feel like it was too "easy" then you're probably approaching it as a type of "cardio." Don't make this mistake.

Change your routine every 4 to 6 weeks. During that time, try different instruments. For example, you could start with your treadmill and then move to your rebounder after a few weeks. Here is a program you can try.

Warm-Up	Set 1		Set 2	
	Exertion	Recovery	Exertion	Recovery
1 min	1 min	2 min	1 min	2 min

Set 3		Set 4		Set 5	
Exertion	Recovery	Exertion	Recovery	Exertion	Recovery
1 min	2 min	1 min	2 min	3 min	2 min

As you can see, the first four sets are just one minute of exertion, so start with a low resistance and give it all you have. Take a break and recover and then get back on the machine for the next set. Turn up the resistance and push yourself. Strive to get your heart rate a little higher than it was last time.

Running either outdoors or on the treadmill works well with this exercise. But, for maximum fat loss, try a stationary bike (or recumbent bike). This will help work the big muscles in your legs. By working the bigger muscle you'll speed up your weight loss.

You could cycle a number of workouts to take you through an entire year. When you eventually come back to this workout, you'll be amazed by how your capacity and recovery times have improved.

What to Do Between Your PACE Workouts

Q: *"Dear Dr. Sears, Is there anything I can do in between my PACE workouts? For example, if I do PACE at the gym three times a week, what can I do on my off days? Would calisthenics work for this? If so, how do you do calisthenics with PACE?"*

A: Calisthenics can build strength, lower your blood pressure, burn fat, relieve many types of lower back pain and improve your chances of staying active and independent as you age.

First, try this simple test: Sit at the end of your chair with your feet flat on the floor. With your hands in your lap, bend from the waist, lean forward and try to stand up. Pump with your legs.

Was that easy or difficult? You may not realize it, but that's the most important movement you have. Compound hip and leg movements work the muscles that keep you mobile. It gets you out of a chair, out of bed, out of a car and up the stairs. Lose that power and you'll be wheelchair bound. Increase it and you'll be moving around until the day you die.

Take the Hindu squat for example:

Here's what you do: Stand with your feet shoulder-width apart. Extend your arms out in front of you, parallel to the ground with your hands open and palms facing down. Inhale briskly and pull your hands straight back. As you pull back, turn the wrists up and make a fist. At the end of the inhalation, your elbows should be behind you with both hands in a fist, palm side up.

From this position, exhale, bend your knees and squat. Let your arms fall to your sides and touch the ground with the tips of your fingers. Continue exhaling and let your arms swing up as you stand. This brings you back to the starting position: standing straight up with your arms extended in front of you, hands open and palms facing down.

Repeat at the pace of one repetition every four seconds. Once you are comfortable with the form, you can increase your speed to one squat per second. Do as many as you can until you become winded and start to pant. Let's say that number is 50.

When you recover to comfortable breathing, do another set of 50. Recover again. During your recovery, shake out your limbs, relax, walk around and drink water if you're thirsty. Then, try another set of 50.

If you can complete three sets of 50 Hindu squats, you will have finished a great PACE workout.

It's not hard to get great results from this routine, but you have to do them. Try doing three sets, three times a week for six weeks. That's my challenge to you. You'll be amazed by the results.

If you can keep up with it, your lung volume will blossom. Your thighs will become rock hard and strong enough for you to pounce. You'll start to fly up stairs and lifting things won't be a problem. Try it.

Drawing a Blank at the Gym?

Q: *"Here's my problem: I don't really know what to do when I get to the gym. I understand the concepts in your book but when I get to the gym and look around at the equipment, I draw a blank."*

A: I understand your situation. It's common for my patients to ask me for a more specific plan for taking PACE into the gym. I have a few suggestions for you…when you get to the gym, just focus on the basics. There are dozens of exercises in your PACE book. But for now, I'll give you just one.

When you're ready to start your workout, follow this checklist:

- Use the routine I give you here.
- On your machine, find a resistance level that's comfortable for you.

As you get started, consider these points:

- <u>Do one thing differently</u>. Think about your last routine… make this routine a little more challenging than the last. You could increase the resistance or you could increase the pace of each exertion period.
- <u>Feel yourself pant</u>. After each exertion period, feel your breath

accelerate as your lungs try to fill the oxygen deficit you just created.

- <u>Recover fully</u>. Get off your machine and walk around. Drink some water. Let your heart rate come down. Feel rested before you start again. Don't worry about how long it takes.

Set 1		Set 2		Set 3	
Exertion	**Recovery**	**Exertion**	**Recovery**	**Exertion**	**Recovery**
4 min	Variable	3 min	Variable	2 min	Variable

You can't go wrong here. If you're not sure where to start, or if you just want a more basic routine to follow, this will work.

Follow the guidelines I mentioned above. Find a resistance level that's challenging but not too hard. Give it all you can during your exertion period and take as long as you need to recover. Don't think too much about it. Just do it and give yourself a challenge.

The next time you do PACE, change one thing. If you want to keep the resistance the same during your first set, fine. But you can turn up the resistance on your second set. You can leave the resistance at the same level for your third set. Or you can turn it up.

Do whatever you need to do to make it different and challenging. Making small changes in the same direction will help you succeed.

Confused About Heart Rate?

Q: *"I'm confused about heart rate… I've read there are different ways to calculate maximum heart rate. Also, once you know what your max heart rate is, what do you do with it? Should you hit your max heart rate every time? There's a big difference between what they* *tell me my max heart rate is and what I can actually achieve during exercise."*

A: Heart rate is a common concern. Let me clarify a few things about heart rate and how best to use it during your PACE routine.

While 220 minus your age is still the easiest and most widely used method to calculate your maximum heart rate, there are other ways. Some of these alternative formulas have interesting clinical studies behind them.

The controversy around the "220 minus your age" formula is that it slightly overestimates the max heart rate for younger people, and slightly underestimates the max heart rate for older people.

Using this formula, a 20-year-old would have a maximum heart rate of 200 (220 – 20 = 200). But this is slightly high. In actuality, a 20-year-old has a max heart rate of about 194. On the other end, a 60-year-old has a max heart rate of 160 based on the "220 minus your age" formula (220 – 60 = 160). But the truth is closer to about 166 for someone that age.

If you want to make the correction, use this formula:

208 – 0.7 (age) = Max heart rate

If you are 60, multiply your age by 0.7 and that gives you 42. Then subtract 42 from 208. That gives you 166.

Now that you've established an upper limit, what does max heart rate mean and what do you do with that number during your PACE routine?

Your max heart rate is a way of measuring your heart's level of conditioning. But just because your max heart is listed as 166 for your age (if you're 60) it doesn't necessarily mean you can get your own heart rate that high.

In practice you may find that you can only get your heart rate to 150. That's not a problem. Consider it your base line – your starting point. As you become more conditioned you'll strive to slowly and gently increase your maximum heart rate knowing that 166 is the normal maximum.

Maximum heart rate is a critical measure of fitness. Your overall *cardiac output* is a combination of stroke volume and maximum heart rate. Stroke volume is how much blood you pump with every beat and your maximum heart rate is the speed at which you can pump that blood.

Heart attacks don't happen because your heart lacks endurance. Heart attacks happen when your cardiac output is too low to handle a stressful situation.

If you find yourself in sudden need of extra oxygen – and your heart lacks the stroke volume and speed required to meet that need – you've just triggered a heart attack.

This can happen when you're lifting something heavy, when you're exercising, when you're being intimate with your partner or if you've just received shocking news about a loved one.

When you challenge your max heart rate during your PACE routine, you're building up your *reserve capacity* – the extra pumping power you need during times of stress. The more reserve capacity you have, the lower your risk of heart attack.

Use your max heart rate as a guide. If you're just starting out, try and establish a base line. Monitor your heart rate during exertion and see how high it goes. Use your PACE program. Try doing three or four sets with recovery in between. By the time you're on your third or fourth set, your heart rate should be climbing to its upper limit. Write it down and keep a log.

As you make progress, slowly increase the challenge. You'll see your max heart rate get higher over time.

Are You Too Old for PACE?

Q: *"My father, who's 71, used to be a runner for years. That was before his hip replacement surgery. Lately he's been trying to get back into an exercise routine, but can't quite seem to find something that works. My own workouts are pretty intense – I do sprints myself – so they're not an option for him. But I'd like to help him out. So my question is, can PACE work for someone his age? And what sort of workout would you recommend?"*

A: I get a lot of questions about whether PACE is too "intense" for people over 65. I can assure you it's not. In fact, some of the program's most ardent fans have to deal with limitations caused by injury or other age-related conditions.

Most people think they have to push themselves hard to get results when they begin working with PACE.

While it's true that your dad will have to focus on intensity levels while exercising, he *won't ever* have to work at uncomfortable levels to get results.

It's a fine point, but one worth clarifying: PACE isn't just about achieving "intensity" for its own sake in order to get in shape.

Quite the opposite in fact: it's about pushing yourself *just a little bit* each time you do it – and then resting.

This definitely does *not* mean pushing yourself too far, too fast. This is why PACE actually works better than conventional training for folks like your dad. When I work with them, I stress that they can and should go at their own "pace."

So let him start at whatever level he's comfortable with. As soon as he starts to pant, he's reached his peak lung capacity, built up an oxygen debt, and he will add to his heart's reserve capacity. He can stop right there.

Then he can rest and recover. Make sure he knows to recover *fully* before he starts up again.

Here's a routine your dad might consider:

Set 1		Set 2		Set 3	
Exertion	**Recovery**	**Exertion**	**Recovery**	**Exertion**	**Recovery**
4 min	Variable	3 min	Variable	2 min	Variable

As far as the right kind of exercise goes, I suggest swimming if he has access to a pool. It's got many of the benefits of resistance training without any of the strain on joints, tendons, or ligaments that comes with sprints or other high-impact routines.

An important point to bear in mind: with swimming, you increase intensity by either swimming faster or going for a longer distance. Again, *the amount of time shouldn't change*, only the intensity.

So your dad can start out doing just one lap, depending on the size of the pool, or even half a lap, and then rest.

It's as easy as that. He'll get the same benefit you're getting without the risk of injury. Who knows? Maybe you can join him to switch things up in your own routine and enjoy a little father/son time together.

Sidestep This Boring Routine for Bigger Muscles

Q: *"Do I have to give up weightlifting to do PACE? I like the way my body looks and I don't really want to lose my muscle. Is there a way I can use weights but still do your program?"*

A: I understand your problem. It's something a lot of weightlifters ask me. Here's my take on weights and PACE.

Weightlifting does give you some benefit, no doubt about it. You're boosting muscle mass and raising your metabolism. Those are good things.

There are two problems I have with weight training (as opposed to *strength* training – more on that in a minute):

1) It's a fundamentally unnatural exercise. Can you think of a single circumstance in nature that would demand you isolate a single muscle group and work it over and over? There really isn't one.

So although you're seeing bigger muscles – and shaping your body in a very specific way – you're also violating the principles your physiology was designed to meet. Over time, this can lead to injury. Your joints, tendons, and ligaments are particularly vulnerable.

2) Because it's so focused on increasing muscle size, you stop focusing on the goal of PACE, challenging your heart and lungs. You want to be sure that you're getting up to a point where your entire cardiovascular system is "maxed out," in the same way that your muscles reach "failure" when you lift weights. And you want to do that repeatedly, with periods of rest in between, over the course of twenty minutes of exertion.

The problem is that if you try to do this while limiting yourself to weights only, I'll bet you'll find it doesn't work. You're only going to put yourself at greater risk of injury, and you won't be able to get that sustained heart pumping action that really gets your fat-burning machine going. (Imagine trying to reach your maximum heart rate doing bicep curls.)

This *doesn't* mean you have to throw out everything you've learned from lifting weights in order to do PACE. In fact there are similarities.

The concepts of "rest-and-repeat" and using resistance are key to both lifting weights and PACE. The difference is that with PACE, you're not isolating just one muscle and taxing it to the max. You're using large muscle groups and exercising them to get your *entire cardiovascular system* to the point of maximum exertion.

These periods of intense exertion are then followed by rest. This is the way your body was designed to work out. It's real "strength training."

The result is that your entire body gets stronger and more efficient over time instead of a single muscle group. This is what I call "functional strength." It's what helps you carry a box of books up five flights of stairs. It's the "get-up-and-go" that gives you stamina throughout the workday.

Take a look at Chapter 9. It talks about this. Try starting out with one of the calisthenic routines and see if it works for you. You can switch to a different routine every two months to rotate muscle groups.

If you want to add a weightlifting element to your routine, you could go with one of the squat routines in your PACE book but maybe hold a set of light weights in both hands (no more than say, 20 lbs). This will give you that familiar "burn" from the extra exertion that you're used to getting during a workout without compromising the PACE approach.

How Can You Make PACE Work for the Long Term?

Q. *"I've probably tried every exercise program under the sun. And I've never been able to stick to any of them. Exercising is just too boring! I went to some of the aerobics classes at the gym. But I feel silly jumping around like that. I don't have time for long routines. How can I be sure I'll stick with PACE?"*

A. I understand that most people hate to work out. And when you perform the same old routines, it gets boring and you give up.

The reason is your body isn't built to do the same thing over and over again. It needs you to change things up. No one gets excited about doing chores. Traditional exercise is just that. A chore. You don't like it, and your body doesn't like it either.

So, the short answer to your question is: Stop doing what bores you! Find exercises that feel more like play than work.

For example, maybe you haven't jumped rope since you were a kid, but it's a fun, quick way to do PACE. You can find good quality jump ropes at your local sporting goods store like Sports Authority or discount store like Wal-Mart for around $15.

To make sure you're getting the right length, stand on the middle of the rope and lift up the handles. They should fit below your arm pits.

For a nice warm-up and to get your rhythm, start jumping rope slowly for about 30 seconds. Then, follow the routine below. Try to increase the number of jumps per exertion period each time.

As always, this isn't set in stone. Modify it to what you like to do. And remember to always go at your own pace, leaving enough time for your body to recover.

Rope Jumping

Warm-Up	Set 1		Set 2	
	Exertion	Recovery	Exertion	Recovery
30 sec	30 sec	1 min	1 min	1 min

Set 3		Set 4		Set 5	
Exertion	Recovery	Exertion	Recovery	Exertion	Recovery
1 min	30 sec	2 min	30 sec	1 min	30 sec

You're Not Seeing Results... What Do You Do?

Q: *"I've been doing your PACE program but I haven't seen any results. I use the equipment at my gym. I have about 20 to 30 pounds to lose but nothing is coming off. I never feel winded like you say. What am I doing wrong? Is there some secret I don't know about?"*

A: The fat busting benefits of PACE are available to everyone. Let's see if there's something you're missing.

Sometimes people practice PACE like it was a traditional cardio routine and that's where you might get into trouble. If you simply start your workout and "watch the clock," you may not get a real PACE workout.

Most of us have built in workout habits and sometimes they get in the way. Clock watching is one of them.

Here's what I mean: Let's say you're on a stationary bike. You set the resistance and off you go. To pass the time you read a magazine while you pedal away. Every so often you look up at the clock on your stationary bike. Two minutes pass… five minutes pass… still not done yet… back to your magazine.

This approach will get you nowhere.

Effective exercise is not like baking a cake. You don't set the clock and then passively wait around until it's done. Most cardio workouts are like this. You set the clock for 40 minutes and then zone out while you read a book or watch one of the TVs mounted above the exercise equipment.

I don't recommend reading while you do your PACE routine. PACE is not passive. It's dynamic and full of intensity. It doesn't take a lot of time but you should "feel the burn."

Here's a PACE checklist. Consider these points as you do your workout:

- **Oxygen Debt:** Do you feel winded after each exertion period? Are you panting? Do you feel like you've pushed yourself?

- **Heart Rate:** Do you notice your heart rate going up slightly after you finish each exertion period? (This is a sign you've achieved oxygen debt.) Are you able to progressively challenge your maximum cardiac output?

- **Recovery:** Do you allow enough time for recovery? During recovery do you get off your instrument and walk around? Do you relax and drink water? Do you focus on your breath, allowing it to become slow and deep?

- **Worthy Challenge:** Do you do the same routine every time, or do you progressively challenge yourself, making sure you do something a little different than before?

- **Diet and Lifestyle:** Do you sabotage your PACE efforts by routinely eating or drinking things that will work against you? PACE will work without changing your diet but if you constantly load up on empty carbs, you'll have a hard time achieving lasting results.

Next time you do PACE, don't watch the clock. Give your heart and lungs a worthy challenge and allow yourself to cool down afterward. Review your checklist and make sure you're hitting every point.

Post-Workout Drinks Help Build New Muscle

Q: *"Should I eat before or after working out? Are there supplements to take?"*

A: These guidelines will help you burn fat faster and get more out of PACE:

Do not eat right before your PACE workout. PACE involves a progressive level of exertion, so it's best to not eat an hour before or after your workout.

After you finish, drink enough water to fill your stomach. Give yourself a little more than you're thirsty for. When you get hungry a little later, go ahead and eat a regular meal.

When I do my PACE routine, I usually follow it up with lots of water. By the time I'm out of the shower and dressed, I'm ready to eat.

Another option is adding protein to your post-exercise drink. You deplete amino acids during a workout and protein powder is a good way of putting them back. But there's more… recent studies show adding protein to a recovery drink reduces muscle damage, and helps rehydration by helping fluids stay in and around your cells.[1]

What's more, added protein will boost your future performance. In one study, cyclists were able to ride 29% longer in their first workout and 40% longer in their second – just from adding a bit of protein into their recovery drink. In the study, they used Gatorade, but I don't recommend it. Gatorade is full of artificial sweeteners. Water with one scoop of protein powder and some berries is better.[2]

For supplements, one of my favorites is another amino acid, L-arginine. It helps with muscle loss, especially as you age.

Muscle loss with aging is something I measure everyday. When I show people they've lost muscle mass, no one is happy about it. Healthy muscles boost your resting metabolism, make you more vigorous and make it easier for you to stay trim.

With L-arginine, you can prevent muscle loss and restore lost muscle. I am familiar with a study showing 5 grams of L-arginine dramatically boosted muscle mass and strength in just 12 weeks. It also reduced body fat.[3]

In the muscle, L-arginine works as a building block for creatine. Your body needs creatine to build and maintain healthy, strong muscles. By helping your body to make more creatine, L-arginine helps you keep your muscles healthy, strong, and lean.

Take up to 5 grams each day. For doses this high, you really have to use a powder. Because L-arginine is an amino acid, proteins compete with its absorption. For this reason, you shouldn't take it with meals. Instead, take it between meals on a relatively empty stomach. Simply take a teaspoon of powder and mix it with water.

Endnotes

1 Seifert JG, Protein added to sports drink improves fluid retention. *Journal of Sports Nutrition and Exercise Meatabolism European* (In Press).

2 Saunders MJ, et al. Effects of a Carbohydrate-Protein Beverage on Cycling Endurance and Muscle Damage. *Medicine & Science in Sports & Exercise*. 2004 Jul;36(7):1233-8.

3 Flakoll P, et al. "Effect of beta-hydroxy-beta-methylbutyrate, arginine, and lysine supplementation on strength, functionality, body composition and protein metabolism in elderly women," *Nutrition* 2004; 20(5): 445-451

APPENDIX C

Research Summaries

CHAPTER 1

Schunemann H, Dorn J, Grant BJ, et al. Pulmonary Function is a Long-term Predictor of Mortality in the General Population. *Chest.* **2000;118(3);656-664.**

1195 adults (554 men and 641 women) aged 20 to 89 years participated in a prospective cohort study. FEV(1) was used to assess pulmonary function at baseline and at 5, 10, 15, 20, and 25-years after enrollment. A sequential survival analysis revealed a significant negative relationship between pulmonary function and all-cause mortality. There was also a significant negative relationship between pulmonary function and ischemic heart disease mortality. Further analysis revealed significantly higher all-cause mortality in the participants in the lowest quintile of pulmonary function relative to participants in the highest quintile of pulmonary function.

Perkins GD, Stephenson B, Hulme J, Monsieurs KG. Birmingham assessment of breathing study (BABS). *Resuscitation.* **2005;64(1): 109-113.**

Forty-eight second-year medical students were shown six video clips depicting normal, abnormal, or absent breathing. The students were asked to indicate whether or not the patient in the video was breathing and whether the breathing was normal or abnormal.

They were also asked to indicate the appropriate emergency action (rescue breathing or recovery position) for each patient. The videos were validated by three emergency practitioners, all of whom correctly identified breathing types and appropriate emergency action. Students correctly identified normal breathing 61% of the time, abnormal breathing 61% of the time, and absent breathing 85% of the time. Correct emergency actions were identified 86% of the time for normal breathing, 51% of the time for abnormal breathing, and 85% of the time for absent breathing. The inability of medical students to reliably differentiate normal from abnormal breathing resulted in a large number of incorrect emergency responses.

Kubzasky LD. Angry breathing: a prospective study of hostility and lung function. *Thorax* 2006;61:863-868.

A prospective cohort study involving 670 men, with an average follow-up of 8.2 years. Hostility was measured using the Cook-Medley Hostility Scale and pulmonary function was measured using FEV1 and FVC. At baseline, men in the high hostility group exhibited significantly lower pulmonary function compared with men in the medium/low hostility group. This effect persisted even after adjusting for smoking and education. Higher hostility was also significantly associated with a more rapid decline in pulmonary function.

CHAPTER 2

Lee IM, Sesso HD, Oguma Y, et al. Relative intensity of physical activity and risk of coronary heart disease. *Circulation*. 2003;107(8):1110-11166.

7337 men (mean age 66 years) were followed for 8-years. Using the Borg Scale, participants were asked to report their perceived level of exertion during exercise (weak, moderate, somewhat strong, strong). 551 men developed CHD during the follow-up period.

Multivariate analysis revealed a significant inverse association between perceived exercise intensity and risk of CHD.

Lee IM, Hsieh CC, Paffenparger RS Jr. Exercise intensity and longevity in men. The Harvard Alumni Health Study. *JAMA*. 1995;273(15):1179-1184.

17,321 Harvard alumni males completed questionnaires regarding their physical activity. Participants were followed for between 22 and 26 years. During the follow-up period, 3728 cases of all-cause mortality were reported. Analysis of the relative risks of death revealed a significant inverse relationship between total physical activity and mortality. Vigorous activity was associated with increased longevity, while non-vigorous activity was not.

Siegel A, Stec JJ, Lipinska I, et al. Effect of Marathon Running on Inflammatory and Hemostatic Markers. *Amer Jour Card*. 2001;88(8):918-920.

Researchers examined the effect of prolonged episodes of physical exercise by examining the effect of marathon running on a variety of hematological variables. Immediately following marathon completion, participants demonstrated significant increases in CRP, vWF, D-dimer, and fibrinolytic activity, and a significant decrease in fibrinogen levels. Platelet studies demonstrated a significantly decreased lag time to aggregation with collagen and an increase with epinephrine. At 24-hours post-race, significant elevations were still observed in D-dimer and vWB levels. The decreased lag time to aggregation also persisted. Hematocrit and red blood cells counts were unchanged immediately post-race, but were significantly decreased at 24-hours post-race. BUN also increased 24-hours post-race, however serum creatinine and electrolytes remained unchanged. The marathon-induced increase in inflammatory markers of cardiac risk, combined with evidence of sub-clinical intravascular coagulation suggest that marathon running mimics the damage often seen in the early stage of cardiac events.

Möhlenkamp S, Lehmann N, Breuckmann F, et al. Running: the risk of coronary events: Prevalence and prognostic relevance of coronary atherosclerosis in marathon runners. *Eur Heart J.* **2008;29(15):1903-1910.**

108 male marathon runners were evaluated with regard to the presence of coronary artery calcification and risk of cardiovascular disease. Data from the runners was compared with age-matched controls and Framingham risk score match controls. Coronary artery calcification in marathon runners was similar to aged-matched controls, but significantly elevated relative to FRS-matched controls. Four runners experienced coronary events during the 21-month follow-up period. The likelihood of remaining coronary-event free was inversely related to the degree of coronary artery calcification.

Neilan TG, Januzzi JL, Lee-Lewandrowski E, et al. Myocardial Injury and Ventricular Dysfunction Related to Training Levels Among Nonelite Participants in the Boston Marathon. *Circulation.* **2006;114(22):2325-2333.**

60 participants in the Boston Marathon participated in a study to assess the potential for cardiac damage during long-distance running. Baseline levels of triponin and N-terminal probrain naturetic peptide (NT-proBNP) were obtained, along with baseline echocardiographic measurements. Pre-race triponin levels were normal in all subjects. Post-race levels were greater than the 99th percentile for 60% of participants, and 40% had triponin levels above the concentration used to diagnose myocardial necrosis. N-terminal probrain levels were approximately doubled post-race. Post-test echocardiographic measurements also revealed significant changes in cardiac function.

Liu M, Bergholm R, Makimattila, S, et al. A marathon run increases the susceptibility of LDL to oxidation in vitro and modifies plasma antioxidants. *Am J Physiol Endocrinol Metab.*1999;276(6 pt 1): E1083-E1091.

Blood samples were collected from 11 runners to determine if participation in a marathon increased the production of oxygen free radicals. Blood was collected prior to the marathon, immediately post-race, and 4-days post race and assayed for the levels of circulating antioxidants and LDL oxidizability *in vitro*. Both immediately post-race and 4-days post-race, an increase in LDL oxidizability was observed, as measured by a reduction in the lag time for formation of conjugated dienes.

Hetland ML, Haarbo J, Christiansen C. Low bone mass and high bone turnover in male long distance runners. *Journal of Clinical Endocrinology & Metabolism.* 1993;77(3):770-775.

120 physically active men (aged 19 – 56) were studied to evaluate the effect of running on bone mass and bone turnover. Measurements of bone mineral content were taken in the lumbar spine, total body, proximal femurs, and forearm. Bone turnover was assessed using urinary pyridinium cross-links, plasma osteoclacin, and serum alkaline phosphatase. An inverse relationship between distance run/week and bone mineral content at all measured sites. In addition, elite runners exhibited a 20 – 30% increase in bone turnover. These data suggest male runners experience accelerated bone loss.

Lee IM, Sesso HD, Paffenparger RS Jr. Physical activity and coronary heart disease risk in men: does the duration of exercise episodes predict risk? *Circulation.* 2000;102(9): 981-986.

7307 men (mean age 66-years) were asked to report both the type and duration of their physical activities. Participants were followed for 5 years, during which 482 developed CHD. After accounting for the total energy expenditure, it was found that, relative to short-duration exercise, longer-duration exercise did not offer any additional protection from CHD provided that total energy expenditure was similar. These findings support the reported benefits of high-intensity, short-duration exercise.

CHAPTER 3

Williams P. Relationships of heart disease risk factors to exercise quantity and intensity. *Arch Intern Med.* 1998;158(3):237-245.

The relationship between exercise amount, exercise intensity, and CHD risk factors was studied in 8896 participants (7059 men, 1837 women). Participants were asked to report their average running amount as well as their running intensity (km/hr) during their best recent 10-K race. Increased intensity was significantly associated with lower blood pressure, lower triglycerides, lower CHOL/HDL ratios, lower BMIs, and lower circumferences of waist, hips, and chest. When examining the effects of distance versus intensity, the researchers found that, for men, intensity had a 13.3 times greater effect on SBP, a 2.8 times greater effect on DBP, and a 4.7 times greater effect on waist circumference. For women, relative to distance, intensity had a 5.7 time greater effect on SBP.

CHAPTER 4

Trappe S, Harber M, et al. Single muscle fiber adaptations with marathon training. *J Appl Physiol,* 101:721-727, 2006.

The muscle fibers of seven marathon runners were assessed to determine the effects of marathon training on muscle fiber size. Biopsies from the gastrocnemius muscle were taken prior to training, after 13-weeks of training, and after 3-weeks of taper. Size, strength, speed, and power were determined for both slow-twitch and fast-twitch muscle fibers. Training resulted in a decrease in the size of both slow-and fast-twitch fibers.

Vanhelder WP, Goode RC, Radomski MW. Effect of Anaerobic and Aerobic Exercise of Equal Duration and Work Expenditure on Plasma Growth Hormone Levels. *Eur J Appl Physiol* **1984;52(3): 255-257.**

Researchers examined growth hormone levels in 5 males before, during, and after aerobic and anaerobic exercise. During aerobic exercise, participants cycled continuously at 100W for 20-minutes. During anaerobic exercise, participants cycled at 285W for 1-minute, followed by 2-mintues of rest, and repeated that cycle 17 times. Growth hormone was significantly higher after anaerobic exercise relative to aerobic exercise.

Tremblay A, Simoneau JA, Bouchard C. Impact of exercise intensity on body fatness and skeletal muscle metabolism. *Metabolism.* **1994;43(7): 814-818.**

27 participants were assigned to complete either a 20-week endurance-training program (ET), with a mean total energy cost of 120.4 MJ or a 15-week high-intensity intermittent-training program (HIIT) with a mean total energy cost of 57.9 MJ. The HIIT resulted in a greater loss of subcutaneous fat relative to the ET program. After controlling for the difference in energy costs between the 2 programs, the effect of the HIIT program on fat loss was 9-times greater than the ET program. Muscle glycolytic enzymes were increased in the HIIT group and decreased in the ET group. Markers for beta-oxidation activity were also elevated in the HIIT group.

Murphy M, Nevill A, Neville C, Biddle S, Hardman A. Accumulating brief walking for fitness, cardiovascular risk and psychological health. *Med Sci Sports Exerc.* **2002; 34(9): 1468-1474.**

Two different walking programs were assessed: the first program (long) consisted of one continuous 30-minute walk per day, and the second program (short) consisted of three 10-minute walks per day. Both programs resulted in significant increases in HDL and significant decreases in triglycerides and total cholesterol. Total body skinfolds, waist circumference, and hip circumference were also decreased in both programs. Both groups reported similar reductions in tension/anxiety. VO_2max decreased in both groups, but the decrease was significantly greater in the short group.

Kraemer WJ, Häkkinen K, Newton RU. Effects of heavy-resistance training on hormonal response patterns in younger vs. older men. *J Appl Physio.l* 1999:87(3) 982-992.

Two groups of men, older (62 years) and younger (30 years), participated in a 10-week periodized strength-power training program. Blood was drawn at baseline and at set post-exercise intervals and was assayed for total testosterone, free testosterone, cortisol, growth hormone, lactate, and ACTH. Insulin-like growth factor and insulin-like growth factor binding protein-3 were also assessed pre- and post-training. Both total and free testosterone were higher in younger men than in older men. Both groups demonstrated significant increases in exercise-induced increases in testosterone, although the effect was more pronounced in the younger men.

Tjønna AE, Lee SJ, Rognmo Ø, Stølen TO, et al. Aerobic interval training versus continuous moderate intensity exercise as a treatment for the metabolic syndrome: a pilot study. *Circulation* 2008;118(4):346-354.

Thirty-two patients with metabolic syndrome were randomly assigned to one of three groups: continuous moderate exercise (CME), aerobic interval training (AIT), both done 3 times a week for 16-weeks, or control. Participants in the CME group exercised at 70% of their highest measured heart rate (Hfmax) and participants in the AIT group exercised at 90% of Hfmax. Both exercise programs resulted in a reduction in arterial blood pressure and body weight. Maximal oxygen uptake was increase significantly more following AIT then CME. In addition, AIT resulted in the removal of significantly more risk factors relative to CME. AIM was also significantly more effective than CME at improving endothelial function, insulin signaling, skeletal muscle biogenesis, and reducing blood glucose, and lipogensis.

CHAPTER 6

Tabata I, Nishimura K, Kauzaki M, et al. Effects of moderate-intensity endurance and high-intensity intermittent training on anaerobic capacity and VO$_2$max. *Med Sci Sports Exerc.* 1996;28(10):1327-1330.

Two experimental protocols were used to assess the effects of different exercise intensities on aerobic and anaerobic energy systems. The first protocol was 6-weeks of moderate-intensity endurance training, and the second was 6-weeks of high-intensity intermittent training. At the end of training, the moderate-intensity endurance training group demonstrated a 5 ml.kg.min-1 increase in VO$_2$max, indicating an improvement in aerobic power. No changes in anaerobic capacity were observed. In contrast, the high-intensity intermittent-training group demonstrated a 7 ml.kg.min-1 increase in VO$_2$max as well as a 28% improvement in anaerobic capacity. These data suggest that while moderate-intensity endurance training can improve aerobic power, only high-intensity intermittent-training can improve both aerobic and anaerobic power.

Burgomaster K, Hughes SC, Heigenhauser GJ, Bradwell SN, Gibala MJ. Six sessions of sprint interval training increases muscle

oxidative potential and cycle endurance capacity. *J Appl Physiol.* **2005; 98(6):1985-1990.**

Eight "recreationally active" adults between 21 and 23 years of age participated in a sprint interval training (SIT) protocol. The protocol consisted of six sessions of SIT (using the Wingate test) over 2 weeks, with 1 to 2 days of rest between each session. Citrate synthase (CS) maximal activity, resting muscle glycogen content, and cycle endurance capacity were assessed at baseline and then again 3-days following completion of the SIT protocol. Significant increases were seen in all three measures; CS maximal activity increased 38%, muscle glycogen content increased 26%, and cycle endurance capacity increased 100%.

Talanian JL, Galloway SD, Heigenhauser GJ, Bonen A, Spriet LL. Two weeks of high-intensity interval training increases the capacity for fat oxidation during exercise in women. *J Appl Physiol.* **2007; 102(4):1439-1447.**

Eight women (22.1 +/- 0.2 years old) participated in 2-weeks of high-intensity aerobic interval training (HIIT), consisting of 10 4-minute sessions at approximately 90% Vo(2 peak), with 2-minutes of rest between intervals. Baseline assessments consisted of a Vo(2 peak) test, a 60-minute cycling trial at 60% Vo(2 peak), and multiple hematological and cardiovascular assessments. HIIT increased Vo(2 peak) by 13%, and resulted in a lower heart rate during the last 30 minutes of the post-HIIT 60-minute cycling trial. Net glycogen use was also decreased during the post-HIIT cycling trial. Exercise whole-body fat oxidation increased by 36%, muscle mitochondrial beta-hydroxyacyl-CoA dehydrogenase increased 36%, citrate synthanse maximal activity increased 20%, and total muscle plasma membrane fatty acid-binding protein content increase 25%.

Praet SF, Jonkers RA, Schep G, et al. Type 2 diabetes patients

respond well to interval training. *European Journal of Endocrinology*. 2008;158(2):163-172.

Obese males (n=11) with type 2 diabetes took part in a combined resistance and interval training exercise program. Subjects trained 3 times per week for 10 weeks. Following completion of the training program, researchers observed a 17% increase in muscle strength and a 14% increase in maximal workload capacity. Significant decreases in arterial blood pressure, daily exogenous insulin requirements, fasting plasma glucose, and non-esterified fatty acid concentrations were also observed post-training.

Laughlin MH, Woodman CR, Schrage WG, Gute D, Price EM. Interval training enhances endothelial function in some arteries that perfuse white gastrocnemius muscle. *J Appl Physiol*. 2004; 96(1):233-244.

Male Sprague-Dawley rats were subjected to interval sprint training (IST). IST consisted of 6 2.5-minute exercise bouts, with 4.5 minutes of rest between each bout and continued 5 days/week for a total of 10 weeks. Endothelium-dependent dilation (EDD), endothelial nitric oxide synthase and/or superoxide dismutase-1 protein was assessed following completion of the IST in both the IST group and the control (sedentary) group. EDD was significantly enhanced in IST rats relative to sedentary rats.

Lindsay F, Hawley JA, Myburgh KH, Schomer HH, Noakes TD, Dennis SC. Improved athletic performance in highly trained cyclists after interval training. *Medicine & Science in Sports & Exercise*. 1996;28(11):1427-1434.

Eight competitive cyclists with a background of moderate-intensity endurance training (BASE) were evaluated to determine the effects of a 4-week high intensity interval training program (HIT). The cyclists replaced approximately 15% of their BASE training with HIT training. HIT consisted of six to eight 5-minute repetitions at 80% of peak sustain power output, with 60-seconds of recovery between bouts. HIT resulted in significant improvements in 40-km time trial performance (TT40) and performance on a timed ride to exhaustion at 150% of perceived power output (TF150). The improvement in TT40 can be attributed to significant increases in absolute and relative power output following HIT.

Helgerud J, Helgerud J, Høydal K, Wang E, et al. Aerobic high-intensity intervals improve VO$_2$max more than moderate training. *Medicine & Science in Sports & Exercise.* **2007;39(4):665-671.**

Researchers evaluated the effects of two different intensities of aerobic endurance training programs with two different high-intensity interval training (HIT) programs. All programs were matched for total work and frequency. Forty male participants (healthy, nonsmoking, moderately trained) were assigned to 1 of 4 groups: 1) long slow distance (70% of HRmax); 2) lactate threshold (85% HRmax); 3) 15/15 interval running (15-seconds of running at 90-95% HRmax, followed by 15-seconds of active resting at 70% HRmax); and 4) 4 x 4 minutes of interval running (4 minutes of running at 90-95% HRmax followed by 3-minutes of active rest at 70% HRmax). HIT resulted in significant increases in VO$_2$max (5.5% increase in the 15/15 group and 7.2% increase in the 4 x 4 group). Stroke volume of the heart was also significantly increased in both HIT groups.

CHAPTER 9

Elefteriades JA, Hatzaras I, Tranquill MA et al. Weight Lifting and Rupture of Silent Aortic Aneurysms. *JAMA.* **2003;290(21): 2803.**

Researchers at Yale University School of Medicine reviewed 5 case studies of acute dissection of the ascending aorta during high-intensity activity. Five patients (aged 19 – 53 years) experienced aortic aneurysms, with the onset of dissection pain occurring during strenuous strength activity. Two of the patients were weight-training, two were doing push-ups, and one was attempting to move a heavy structure. None of the patients had a history of hypertension, collagen-vascular disease, or Marfan syndrome. One patient had a family history of aortic disease.

Hatzaras I, Tranquilli M, Coady M, et al. Weight Lifting and Aortic Dissection: More Evidence for a Connection. *Cardiology.* **2007;107(2):103-106.**

Thirty-one cases of aortic dissection during strenuous exercise were studied by researchers at Yale University. The patients consisted of 30 males and 1 female with an average age of 47.3 years (range 19 – 76 years). The dissection was fatal in 10 patients (32.2%). Twenty-seven cases (87%) occurred in the ascending aorta. Only 3 patients (9.7%) had a family history of aortic disease. Based on these findings, the researchers proposed that all individuals who engage in intense strength training get routine echocardiographic screenings.

CHAPTER 10

Cordain L, Miller JB, Eaton SB, et al. Plant-animal subsistence ratios and macronutrient energy estimations in worldwide hunter-gatherer diets. *Am J Clin Nutr.* **2000; 71(3): 682-692.**

Using ethnographic data, researchers determined that hunter-gather populations received a larger portion (45 – 65%) of energy from animal food. Additionally, they determined that 73% of hunter-gatherer societies around the world obtained >50% of their energy from animal food. In contrast, only 14% of hunter-gather societies obtained >50% of their energy from plants. These data demonstrate diets with a relatively high (19 – 35%) of energy from protein.

Wolf RL, Cauley JA, Baker CE, et al. Factors associated with calcium absorption efficiency in pre-and perimenopausal women. *Am J Clin Nutr.* **2000;72(2): 466-471.**

Calcium absorption was assessed in 142 pre- and perimenopausal women. Factors found to have a significant positive effect on calcium absorption included: body mass index, dietary fat intake, serum 1,25 dihydroxy vitamin D concentrations, and parathyroid hormone concentrations. Significant inverse associations included: dietary fiber intake, alcohol consumption, physical activity, and symptoms of constipation. Women in the bottom tertile of dietary fat to fiber had 19% lower calcium relative to women in the upper tertile.

Venkatraman JT, Leddy J, Pendergast D. Dietary fats and immune status in athletes: clinical implications. *Med Sci Sports Exer.* **2000 Jul;32(7Suppl):S389-395.**

Low-fat diets (15% fat) have been shown to increase inflammatory immune factors and increase anti-inflammatory immune factors. Low-fat diets have also been shown to negatively affect antioxidant levels and cholesterol ratios. These negative effects can be reversed by increasing dietary fat intake to 32%.

Hunninghake DB, Maki KC, Kwiterovich PO Jr, Davidson MH, Dicklin MR, Kafonek SD. Incorporation of Lean Red Meat into a National Cholesterol Education Program Step I Diet: A Long-Term, Randomized Clinical Trial in Free-Living Persons with Hypercholesterolemia. *J Am Coll Nutr.* **2000;19(3): 351-360.**

The impact on red meat consumption on lipoprotein concentrations was evaluated in 145 hypercholesterolemic men and women. Participants were assigned to begin the study in one of two groups: lean red meat (beef, veal, and pork) or lean white meat (poultry and fish). Diets were followed for 36 weeks, followed by a 4-week washout period during which participants were allowed to eat any type of meat. Participants were then assigned to the alternative group. There were no differences in lipoprotein concentrations between the lean red meat or lean white meat phases of the study. Total cholesterol and LDL levels decreased significantly in both groups, while HDL levels rose in both groups.

Gutierrez M, Akhavan M, Jovanovic L, Peterson CM. Utility of a Short-Term 25% Carbohydrate Diet on Improving Glycemic Control in Type 2 Diabetes Mellitus. *J Am Coll Nutr.* **1998;17(6):595-600.**

Twenty-eight subjects with type 2 diabetes, either treated with diet alone (n=9) or with second generation sulfonylurea agents (n=19) were placed on a low-carbohydrate diet (25% carbohydrate). The diet of each participant was also tailored to their ideal body weight. All oral hypoglycemic agents were discontinued prior to beginning the diet. Following 8-weeks of the low-carbohydrate diet, participants were switched to a diet consisting of 55% carbohydrates. Calories remained consistent across both diets. After the low-carbohydrate phase, all subjects showed significant improvements in fasting blood glucose values and hemoglobin A1c levels. Additionally, participants who had previously been on oral hypoglycemic medications exhibited a significant decrease in weight and diastolic blood pressure. A significant rise in hemoglobin A1c levels was observed when participants followed the 55% carbohydrate diet.

Petzke KJ, Elsner A, Proll J, Thielecke F, Metges CC. Long-Term High Protein Intake Does Not Increase Oxidative Stress in Rats. *J Nutr.* **2000;130(12): 2889-2896.**

The effect of adequate protein (13.8%), moderate protein (25.7%) or high protein (51.3%) diets was examined to determine if high protein intake was a factor in oxidative stress. Hematological markers of oxidative stress, plasma protein carbonyl concentrations, lipid liver peroxide levels, reduced glutathione levels, and leucine kinetics were all assessed. In contrast to the researchers' original hypothesis, the high protein diet did not increase oxidative stress. Additionally, the data suggest a possible relationship between an adequate protein diet and increased oxidative stress.

CHAPTER 11

Rasmussen BB, Tipton KD, Miller SL, et al. An oral essential amino acid-carbohydrate supplement enhances muscle protein anabolism after resistance exercise. *J Appl Physiol*. 2000;88(2): 386 - 392.

Following resistance exercise, six subjects were randomly assigned to consume a drink containing essential 6 grams of amino acids and 35 grams of sucrose or a flavored placebo. The drinks were consumed on 2 different occasions, either 1- or 3-hours after exercise. Leg muscle protein kinetics were assessed via infusion of ring-(2)H(5)-phenylalanine, femoral arterial and venous blood, and muscle biopsies. Phenylalanine net balance and muscle protein synthesis increased relative to pre-drink levels, as well as compared to placebo. These effects were observed at both 1-hour and 3-hour post drink.

Hope BK, Baker R, Edel ED, et al. An overview of the salmonella enteritidis risk assessment for shell, egg, and egg products. *Risk Analysis* 2002;22(2): 203-218.

Of the 69 billion eggs produced each year, researchers estimate that 2.3 million eggs are contaminated with salmonella enteritidis (SE). SE is estimated to cause approximately 661,633 human illnesses per year. Of those, 94% will recover without medical care. Approximately 0.5% are hospitalized and 0.05% result in death. Commercially pasteurized eggs contribute a negligible contribution to SE.

Li Z, Xi X, Gu M, et al. A stimulatory role for cGMP-dependent protein kinase in platelet activation. *Cell* **2003;112(1):77-86.**

Researchers at the University of Illinois College of Medicine proposed that sildenafil (Viagra), via its ability to increase levels of cGMP, has the potential to increase platelet aggregation. This effect was biphasic, with the initial response being enhanced aggregation, followed by an inhibitory phase during which thrombi size was limited.

CHAPTER 12

Dardik IJ. The Origin of Disease and Health: Heart Waves – the Single Solution to Heart Rate Variability and Ischemic Preconditioning; *Cycles.* **1996;46(3):67-79.**

A review of the risks associated with a reduction in heart rate variability (HRV). Retrospective examination of the effects of reduced HRV revealed that reduced HRV is associated with increases in infant mortality, sudden-infant death syndrome, coronary artery disease, multiple sclerosis, type-2 diabetes, as well as all-cause mortality.

Resources

PACE Revolution
www.pacerevolution.com

Al Sears, MD
www.alsearsmd.com

The Wellness Research Foundation
www.wellnessresearch.org

Primal Force
www.primalforce.net

Glycemic Index
www.alsearsmd.com/glycemic-index

American Academy of Anti-Aging Medicine
www.worldhealth.net

American College of Sports Medicine (ACSM)
www.acsm.org

American College for the Advancement in Medicine (ACAM)
www.acam.org

American Council on Exercise
www.acefitness.org

Framingham Heart Study
www.framinghamheartstudy.org

Jonathon Wright, MD
www.tacoma-clinic.com

Jeffry S. Life, MD, PhD
www.drlife.com

Coach Yari
www.getfitin6.com/pace

Jonny Bowden
www.jonnybowden.com

John Defendis
www.defendis.com

How to Get the Most Out of PACE

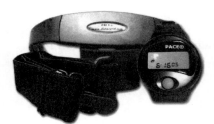

Congratulations on being part of the PACE Revolution.

Measuring your heart rate is critical to the success of PACE. Your heart rate gives a clear and accurate picture of your progress. It helps you …

- **Track Recovery Time.** Your recovery time is a marker for your heart health. If your heart rate doesn't slow down at least 30 beats in the first minute, you're in poor shape. If it slows down more than 50 beats in the first minute, you're in excellent shape.

- **Gauge the Intensity of Your Exertion.** Measuring intensity is an important aspect of your PACE workouts. Underperform and you won't get the benefits. Overperform and you'll put yourself at risk.

- **Determine Whether You've Entered the "Supra-Aerobic Zone."** When you finish an exertion period and go into a recovery period, your heart rate should go up a few ticks. This usually takes place in the first 10 to 15 seconds. As your recovery period continues, your heart rate will start to come down. This is a sure-fire way to know you're doing PACE correctly and will help you build a bulletproof heart and powerful lungs.

Using a heart rate monitor makes it much easier to track your heart rate than stopping to count pulse beats.

This easy-to-use heart rate monitor has everything you need to gauge your exertion levels and find out if you're reaching your supra-aerobic zone. In fact, it has three different audible alarms (two visual alarms) that help you track your progress.

It's durable, lightweight, and comes with a chest strap and wristwatch. This is the best kind, because the chest strap rests right up against your heart, so you know you're always getting an accurate reading. All you have to do is look at your wrist, and everything you need to know is right there on your easy-to-read monitor. It's as simple as that.

Call 866.792.1035 or visit www.pacerevolution.com/hrm

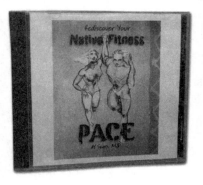

Getting Lean Is as Easy as Pushing Play

Dr. Sears takes you step-by-step through PACE, giving you an insider's look at the revolutionary exercise program that put aerobics out of business.

In this hour-long video, Dr. Sears and his team of fitness experts guide you through the techniques that make PACE work and how to do them. You'll discover the PACE fat burning secrets and see them in practice.

Applied to actual workouts you can do yourself, you'll see the PACE principles laid out in front of you. It's as easy as inserting the DVD and following along. No more guesswork… no more wondering if you're doing it right… You'll get the whole story in a way that's easy to understand and easy to do.

Hearing Dr. Sears explain PACE in his own words gives you an instant sense of recognition. And when you combine his instruction with an actual demonstration of some of his best techniques, everything falls into place. The ease and simplicity becomes clear. If you ever had trouble following PACE, this will wipe out any confusion.

We've been conditioned to believe that burning fat is hard work that takes hours to achieve. But compared to cardio or aerobics, PACE is easy and takes up much less of your time.

PACE is fast and to the point. It's not the grueling drudgery you may be used to... it's not at all what cardio feels like. You feel invigorated after it's done, not tired and bored.

Aside from hearing Dr. Sears explain PACE in his own words, you'll get sample PACE routines for both indoors and out. If you don't have access to a gym, it's not a problem. You'll find a PACE program that fits your needs.

Call 866.792.1035 or visit www.pacerevolution.com/pacedvd

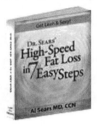

Burn Fat Without Dieting or Counting Calories

Dr. Sears busts the biggest fat-loss lies in **High-Speed Fat Loss in 7 Easy Steps**.

Learn why:

- Counting calories won't help you lose weight
- Eating fat won't make you fat
- Traditional exercise won't keep you lean and trim

High-Speed Fat Loss in 7 Easy Steps returns you to your native diet and makes hitting your ideal weight a sure thing.

Dr. Sears uses these same techniques to slim down his patients. With amazing results… Many patients make double-digit drops in their first month: 12, 18 even 22 lbs. of fat loss in the first 30 days!

Within minutes you'll put these easy-to-understand principles to work and effectively burn fat – even if nothing has worked for you in the past.

Call 866.792.1035 or visit www.pacerevolution.com/flb

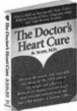

Clinically-Proven Plan of Breakthrough Health Secrets Helps You Build a Powerful, Disease-Free Heart

Dr. Sears' bestselling book, **The Doctor's Heart Cure**, shows you how to stop heart attacks and strokes in a way that's easy to understand and simple to follow. You'll learn how to determine your own risk and put together a program that fits your own needs.

Don't leave yourself vulnerable to the lightning fast and deadly strike of a heart attack or stroke. **The Doctor's Heart Cure** lowers your risk to zero.

Call 866.792.1035 or visit www.pacerevolution.com/dhcb

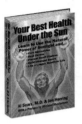

Put One of the Most Dangerous Myths of Our Time to Rest

Your Best Health Under the Sun, gives you everything you need to enjoy the sun safely, while using its power to prevent disease, burn fat and power up your sex life…

Here's a glimpse of what you'll discover:

- How 20 minutes in the sun can prevent 17 deadly cancers
- The 7 dangerous chemicals in sunscreen that increase your risk of skin cancer
- Why skin cancer rates are skyrocketing in cities that get the least amount of sunshine
- The little-known secret that powers-up your sex drive and boosts your sex hormones by an amazing 200%…

How sunlight controls your blood sugar, improves your response to insulin and helps you burn fat…

There is no need to feel guilty, stressed out or worried sick when you are in your native sun… **Your Best Health Under the Sun** gives you an easy-to-follow guide for taking full advantage of the sun's disease-fighting power. And best of all, you'll feel better almost immediately!

Call 866.792.1035 or visit www.pacerevolution.com/sun

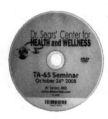

Switch on Your "Immortality" Gene

There's a hidden switch in every cell of your body. It controls how long you live… and when you die. It has the power to extend life—maybe indefinitely.

Most doctors have never heard of it. A group of scientists stumbled upon it just ten years ago. They watched in awe as generation after generation of cells multiplied … without aging.

For the first time ever, you can slow down and even reverse aging.

You'll be in the front row as Dr. Sears and a team of leading anti-aging experts walk you through the process in his brand-new DVD.

Call 866.792.1035 or visit www.pacerevolution.com/ta65

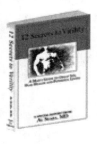

Attention Men: Have More Sex… More Ambition… More Gusto… Stronger Muscles…Bigger Dreams…

Fact: Many modern chemicals closely resemble estrogen. These hormone look-a-likes get into your body and send powerful and confusing messages to your tissues and organs. <u>They can feminize your body and wreak havoc on your sex life</u>.

That's not all: Loss of muscle, ambition and sex drive will zap your enjoyment of life.

But here's the good news…

You Can Get on the Fast Track to *Super* Manhood – Today!

Dr. Sears' book – *12 Secrets to Virility* – exposes the dangers of estrogen and gives you quick and powerful ways to:

- **Toss Your Viagra in the Trash:** Dr. Sears' Simple 2-Step Strategy for Turbo-Charging Your Sexual Performance Will Keep You Rock Hard and Ready for Action – No Matter What Your Age.

- **Eat the Foods You Love – Guilt Free:** Stop Torturing Yourself with Low-Fat "Health Food." Dr. Sears Shows You How to Enjoy Your New York Strip and Improve Your Heart Health at the Same Time.

- **Live Pain Free:** Jump out of Bed, Run to the Store, Walk a Round of Golf… You'll Use the Quick and Easy Solutions that Slash Your Risk of Arthritis and Wipe Out Joint Pain Forever.

Never again will you have to listen to a doctor tell you, "It's just part of the aging process…" *12 Secrets to Virility* will reveal the real truth about male health and aging.

More importantly, the secrets you will learn will transform you. You'll lose your gut, strengthen your body and regain youthful sexuality. Starting as soon as you begin practicing the secrets in *12 Secrets to Virility…*

Call 866.792.1035 or visit www.pacerevolution.com/12sec

Give Your Brain the Power of Total Recall and Extreme Alertness

REPAIR YOUR AGING BRAIN in Just 15 Minutes a Day

FREE REPORT

M.D.

As you age, your mental functions slow down. Both your thinking and your reaction time slow. It's probably natural. But is it unavoidable?

Despite what you may have heard, cognitive decline is not inevitable. What's more, maintaining your memory has little to do with genetics, and even less to do with drugs.

In this report, you'll discover a different approach. It's the best way to improve your mental performance and stave off age-associated cognitive decline. And, it's free!

Many of these simple exercises take just minutes a day. They're easy to understand and easy to do.

You'll find:

1. Tools you can use to reverse cognitive decline

2. How to beat the brain-destroying effects of cortisol

3. The best way to protect yourself from dreaded Alzheimer's disease

Think of your brain as a dynamic system. The neurons respond to environmental factors and mental stimulation. By stimulating your mind, you preserve your memory, and can even restore the clarity you had in your youth!

Research shows the more you use your brain, the less your risk of Alzheimer's. The more connections, or synapses, you can develop between brain cells, the more resistant they are to the disease.

How do you create these connections?

Discover now in Dr. Sears' Free Report – *Repair Your Aging Brain... in Just 15 Minutes a Day!* Get your FREE report INSTANTLY... along with the latest health news and little-known health solutions that really work.

Simply sign up to receive Dr. Al Sears' FREE Health Confidential e-letter, (published 5x per week), plus access to over 420 articles on the HOT topics that affect YOUR health, and we'll immediately send you his exclusive research report... Absolutely FREE!

Call 866.792.1035 or visit www.pacerevolution.com/rybreport

NOTES

NOTES